Losing Weight for Life:

Eating What You Like with the RMR Diet

Losing Weight for Life:

Eating What You Like with the RMR Diet

Fred Civish

CFI
Springville, Utah

ISBN 13: 978-1-59955-165-4

Published by CFI, an imprint of Cedar Fort, Inc., 2373 W. 700 S., Springville, UT 84663
Distributed by Cedar Fort, Inc., www.cedarfort.com

LIBRARY OF CONGRESS CATALOGING-IN-PUBLICATION DATA

Civish, Fred M.
  Losing weight for life : eating what you like with the RMR diet / Fred M.
Civish, Jr.
    p. cm.
  ISBN 978-1-59955-165-4
  1. Low-carbohydrate diet. 2. Reducing diets. 3. Weight loss. 4.
Metabolism. I. Title.

  RM237.73.C52 2008
  613.2'5--dc22

      2008028104

Cover design by Jen Boss
Cover design © 2009 by Lyle Mortimer
Edited and typeset by Heidi Doxey

Printed in the United States of America

10 9 8 7 6 5 4 3 2 1

Printed on acid-free paper

Contents

Introduction

During the Great Depression there was a boy so underweight, his mother took him to the doctor. I was that boy, and the problem was not that there wasn't sufficient food. Dad provided well for us, and Mom was proud of this fact. In the first grade she'd wave my hair, put me in a shirt, tie, and small suit, and then send me to school each day. Heaven forbid I should play in the school yard with other kids. The first time I did this and came home dirty, I learned that lesson. When she got me to the doctor, he took one look at me, reached out, and mussed up my wavy hair and turned to Mom. "Get him out of that suit and tie. Put him in a plaid shirt and corduroys. Send him to school like a normal kid so he can play. Whatever his favorite food is, feed it to him three times a week, and let him eat as much of it as he wants."

I chose macaroni drenched with canned tomatoes. It was, after all, the Great Depression and my choices were somewhat limited.

Within a very few months I progressed from underweight to chubby. From then on in life, I have had a weight problem. Every major weight loss diet I've been on worked—for a while. Then it was back to not weighing myself because I didn't want to know how much weight I was gaining. When I was in my twenties and early thirties, I weighed around 230 pounds.

But as my age progressed, so did my top weights. Finally, by my fifties, each time I went off a diet, my pants size got bigger and bigger. By the time my pants size reached forty-eight, I knew I'd better bite the bullet and get back on the scale. As I knew it would, the scale showed I was back up to within a pound or two of 300 pounds.

I was ashamed to go out in public. I was unable to do the activities I loved such as swimming or walking, and I was depressed. My knees and hips began bothering me and doing almost anything was a strain.

My choices were simple: do nothing and probably die because of it, or lose weight once again. As a result, I have been on nearly every new diet that has come down the pike. I've done fasts lasting from five to seventeen days. Strangely, I found it easier to not eat than to quit dieting once I started. I even did a juice fast lasting six weeks.

In all this, I learned two great lessons. The first was that no diet I ever tried got me to where I really wanted to be or even kept off the weight I'd lost. Whatever it took to permanently lose weight on a diet was lacking in me.

During the last decade or so, I'd generally feel forced to do something when my weight was between 250 and 270 pounds. When my weight finally got up to 278, I firmly decided I would make a life change and only eat every other day. It worked for over a year and I slowly lost weight. I got down to 247, but then, even if I fasted, I stopped losing weight. My body had adjusted to my caloric needs and was matching my metabolism, so I was stuck at that weight.

During all these efforts, I was down to around 200 pounds a number of times and 225 frequently. It was at these times that I learned the second lesson. I learned the tremendous benefits of weighing less. At two hundred pounds, I was not ashamed of such things as being seen out walking the dogs or wearing a swimming suit for regular swims. My knees and hips lost all their pain. I had far more energy to do the other things life requires of us, and the things I did with this extra energy were far easier to accomplish. My feelings of self-worth increased greatly. I didn't have to worry so much about what all that extra weight was doing to my health and body.

There are literally hundreds of sources to verify the health risks of being overweight.[1] These risks include diabetes, coronary heart disease, high blood cholesterol, stroke, hypertension, gallbladder disease, osteo-arthritis (degeneration of cartilage and bone of joints), sleep apnea and other breathing problems, and some forms of cancer (breast, colorectal, endometrial, and kidney). Obesity is also associated with complications of pregnancy, menstrual irregularities, hirsutism (presence of excess body and facial hair), stress incontinence (urine leakage caused by weak pelvic floor muscles), psychological disorders like depression, increased surgical risk, and increased mortality.

Since I've known about these risks for decades and suffered from some of them, is it any wonder I needed to find some way to not only lose weight, but keep it off? Both my mental, emotional, and physical health depended on accomplishing just that.

Then I discovered the RMR diet.

I am neither a doctor nor a dietician. This book is based on my experiences and study through years of diets. You should consult your own physician before trying it.

NOTES

1. One of the best sources I've found online to give a quick but complete overview is the federally sponsored Weight-control Information Network (WIN). By clicking on the various options almost every weight loss problem can be found. A complete copy of their research can also be obtained by phone, toll free: 1-877-946-4627. Or visit their website: http://win.niddk. nih.gov/

1

The Five Building Blocks

Unlike other diets that writers and researchers have made complicated beyond understanding, there are five—and only five—building blocks to make the RMR diet work. If you do these, you will lose weight. Don't do them, and this will probably be just another diet that didn't work for you.

Building Block One: Determine your RMR.

Building Block Two: Calculate the calories in all the servings of the foods you eat.

Building Block Three: Eat up to, or nearly up to, your allotted number of calories each day.

Building Block Four: Snack often.

Building Block Five: You decide what you will do, and not do, to make this diet work for you in the easiest and most successful way possible.

In the rest of this book you will find little tricks to make your diet more effective and help you understand why this diet works so well. It will point out things that make dieting difficult, and what to do about them. You will also read about some of my experiences on the plan. But in all the rest of this book, make Building Block Five part of all you do!

Not everything about this diet is new. Some of it includes the best and most recent information on losing weight and keeping it off. However, it is a diet based on a new principle (RMR). An extremely important part of the diet is making lifestyle changes that will improve your health while helping you burn fat and keep it off for the rest of your life. It is not only by far the most successful fat burning program I have ever been on, but the easiest and least stressful as well.

Whether you know it or not, you are on a metabolic diet. There is no other possibility. Further, you will be on one as long as you live. On this metabolic diet, you are either adding weight, stabilized at a given weight, or losing weight. After all, diet refers to the amount and type of food you eat, not to a weight loss eating plan. Whether you are familiar with it or not, understanding your metabolism is the key to losing weight and maintaining your weight once you've lost some.

Metabolic refers to metabolism, which is simply the amount of energy your body burns under given circumstances. There are only three basic kinds. The first is your Basal Metabolic Rate (BMR). This is the average amount of calories your body burns during the day, given your age, height, weight, and level of physical activity.

Next is your Resting Metabolic Rate (RMR). That is the amount of calories your body burns if you were to sleep twenty-four hours a day. This is based on the same things, excluding your activity rate, because you would be resting, and thus you would not have any activity. The third metabolic rate is the amount of calories your body burns when you have cut your food consumption down to the point where you are literally starving; this is your Starvation Metabolic Rate (SMR).

Knowing your BMR is important because if you are consuming more calories than your BMR, you are putting on fat, if you are matching it, your weight is stabilized, and if you are consuming fewer calories you're burning fat. Nothing new here. It is just a way to measure how your body is reacting to the amount of calories you eat.

Now comes the second kid on the scene, your RMR. This one has changed my life in ways I only dreamed about before. Eating the amount of calories that matches your RMR is what is required to run the machine and maintain your health. Once you know the caloric value of that, you need only eat enough food to match it, and you will burn fat. Why do you burn fat if you match your RMR? Because you are only taking in enough calories to sustain you while you're resting, meaning your body must burn fat to get the energy for every single thing you do when you are not resting. That includes activities such as standing up or walking to the bathroom.

My experience with this diet has been that it is not only the most successful diet I have ever been on, but the easiest as well. The root word for *easiest* is *ease*. When you look up *ease* in a good dictionary, you will see it is defined as contentment or comfort, whether of body or mind; freedom from pain, trouble or annoyance of any kind; or tranquility. The vagaries and events in our lives do not allow complete ease with almost anything, so an easy fat-burning program is especially appealing.

Above all, however, once I was on this plan for a short while I came to the realization that it is the kind of eating I can live with for the rest of my life. I am not alone in our society when it comes to losing weight often and regaining it all (or more) just as often. "Various studies have suggested that, on average, four years after starting to lose weight, people have gained at least three-quarters of it back."[1] Generally speaking, within five years of losing weight, only five percent of people have kept it all off.

So two things are at work here. Now, we cannot only achieve the weight of our dreams, but by following this plan, we can obtain all the mental and health benefits of being at an appropriate weight for our gender and age.

How did I come upon this marvelous, easy to accomplish, satisfying eating plan? My step-daughter Kim began losing weight. I asked her how she was doing it, and she said it was something new the physical trainer at her place of employment had shown her. I was intrigued, but then I'd been on these fad diets before. Then my other step-daughter and my wife, Bobbie, both began losing weight following Kim's advice. Bobbie tried to tell me a number of times how different and easy this diet was. In effect, I told her that was nice and hoped she'd have a lot of luck with it.

It was around this same time that the weight I had been losing by fasting every other day began to level off. My body had learned how to deal with the way I was eating and would match my metabolism to my food intake over time. The scale showed me I'd reached an impasse.

I can't express the discouragement it brought me to fast every other day and still not lose weight. It had taken tremendous willpower to set that plan into my life, and I was resigned to eating that way from now on. At least I had been resigned until I stopped losing weight. What to do? Start eating every day and once again put back all I'd lost? Or go on at the same weight (248 pounds) by starving myself every other day?

I got Kim to outline the easy-to-follow steps for me, began following them, and lost weight the first week. Then I began to research the diet and found that the only direct reference I could find on it was hardly helpful at all.[2] All it did was describe what a wonderful thing the diet was. But every diet I have ever read about has those descriptions.

I clicked on some of the site's suggested links and found one site where you could purchase a number of electronic items, and on another you could register yourself on the diet for twenty dollars.

Now, more than sixty pounds lighter, without having to register, with much more study and personal experience on how to do it, I feel it is time a good book on the subject was available for everyone who has suffered as I have with being obese.

WHY WE NEED THE RMR DIET

That the American population is becoming grossly obese is not a new concept, nor can we escape regular items about this trend on TV and in the papers. For example, Jay Leno frequently starts obesity jokes with the line, "How fat are we getting when . . ."

The Center for Disease Control has stated, "In 2007 only one state (Colorado) had a prevalence of obesity less than 20 percent. Thirty states had a prevalence equal to or greater than 25 percent; three of these states (Alabama, Mississippi and Tennessee) had a prevalence of obesity equal to or greater than 30 percent."[3]

What isn't so well covered or realized is that these disturbing trends are only about those considered obese, not simply overweight. The distinction between being obese and just overweight depends on one's gender, height, and weight. All of this is easily computed by using the various sources for determining one's Body Mass Index (BMI). For a calculator or a simple chart type "calculating BMI" into your search engine.

And the problem is getting even worse. Not only is it plaguing adults, but children as well. In addition, the higher your BMI, the more likely you are to be plagued by the many health problems associated with being overweight. It is generally accepted that a BMI of less than 18.5 is considered underweight, 18.5 to 24.9 is normal, 25 to 29.9 is overweight (fat) and a BMI of 30 or greater is considered obese.

Most troubling, it seems, is the general attitude of those who are not so afflicted when they see pictures of grossly obese people walking with their fat jiggling behind them as they move. The word *slob* comes to mind. But however most people define it, it is never complimentary and generally includes the thought that those who are fat are somehow deficient as people or they would not let themselves get in such bad shape.

This attitude is so prevalent that most of us with weight problems also feel that way about ourselves. I knew I was strong and had ample willpower, but darn it, I just couldn't seem to solve my weight problem—until the RMR diet. Having such faith in myself, I also had faith that others were just as unable to really help themselves no matter what they tried.

HOW THE RMR DIET WORKS

If there was only the problem of not eating so much, it would be a cinch to lose weight. Unfortunately, that is only one small part of the problem. There are many other impediments to losing weight that range from emotional eating to genetics.

So how does the RMR eating plan help all this? Perhaps the most important factor for me was that my RMR was high enough in calories that I could eat far more than I had on any other diet and still lose weight. In fact, although my RMR was around eighteen hundred calories to start, after the first couple of weeks I cut my daily intake down to around fifteen hundred. I didn't really need all that food, and even at fifteen hundred calories daily I was satisfied and rarely felt anything even close to hunger pangs.

Another important part of the plan is that you should eat at least two regular meals, minimum, preferably three, and frequent snacks are a must. By "eating smaller more frequent meals, going no longer than three hours without food . . . you prevent your body from slowing down your metabolism."[4] Add to this the fact that there are absolutely no restrictions on the type of food one can eat, and it hardly seems like a diet at all. I can eat what I've always eaten and enjoy it. Anytime I feel anything even close to a hunger pang, I can snack. And my scale is dropping slowly but regularly. Given all this, the only real change in my life is that I had to begin measuring everything I ate, calculating its caloric value, and logging it in every day to make sure I didn't go over my limit.

Determining your RMR is easy. Before continuing, however, it needs to be clear that whether we're talking about BMR, RMR, or SMR, no one can get more than a close approximation. There are three different ways to compute RMR, for example, and all give different caloric amounts. The one I recommend is an online version from Shape Up America. By typing in your height, weight, age, and sex, the calculator figures out your RMR for you. This particular calculator is important, because other calculators I've used vary significantly. One even said my RMR was as high as 2,450 calories.[5] Whichever calculator you use, in the end it will be the scales that let you know if you are eating the right amount of calories.

As dangerous as it is to our health to eat too many calories for long periods of time, an even greater danger is not getting enough. That is starvation, and, as was mentioned, the metabolic name for that is SMR. Eating only enough calories to match this metabolic rate is far more dangerous to your health, and the problems from doing so surface far more quickly than those that result from being obese.

Depending on the individual, starvation begins when your caloric intake reaches about fifty percent of your BMR. That means if your BMR is twenty-two hundred calories, you could go into the starvation mode on a diet that restricted you to less than eleven hundred calories per day. Again, however, the exact effect on caloric intake and the starvation mode is only an approximation. You can determine the level of calories at which your body might begin going into starvation mode by calculating your BMR and dividing it in half.

There is considerable controversy about SMR and diet programs. Most of that is because some people have thought a day or two below one thousand calories would trigger it. This is not true; starvation mode occurs only after considerable time below the needed calories to sustain RMR.[6]

Another misconception is that when you go into the starvation mode, your body stops losing fat. One article notes, "Many fear that going into starvation mode will drastically reduce their metabolic rate and cause them to hoard calories and gain weight instead of losing." This same article then goes on to detail a Minnesota Study in which men were fed on a semi-starvation diet of significantly less than their " 'normal' maintenance calories." The article then asserts that "at no point did the men stop losing fat until they hit 5 percent body fat at the end of the study." However, with regard to the dangers of the starvation mode, this same article went on to say, "Did the Minnesota men suffer negative consequences from the experience? They most certainly did, and, interestingly, many of the same consequences that anorexics experience."[7]

Another source claims, "Going on a 'crash' diet where you severely restrict your calories is harmful because your body goes into a 'starvation' mode metabolically. This causes a number of negative side effects. One of these is that your body will break down proteins from your muscle tissue to use as fuel." The source concludes with the following information, "But can it cause brain damage? Yes. It can also cause liver failure, kidney failure, stroke, depression and lead to eating disorders like anorexia and bulimia."[8]

Another article on this subject says, "The mind and the body are inextricably linked, and never is this more apparent than when you go on a diet. . . . Suddenly, you may find yourself clipping recipes, planning menus, cooking elaborate meals or dishes for others (neither of which you'll eat yourself), or even dreaming about food at night. . . . Suddenly, you develop the urge and the capacity to binge, and you no longer feel satisfied after eating what you used to consider a normal meal."[9]

Often, when you are in the starvation mode you don't even know it. That is why knowing the symptoms is important. I can testify to the insidiousness of this based on my own experiences with low calorie diets in the past.

Regarding clipping recipes (or searching for them on the Internet) when one is in the starvation mode, I have literally thousands of recipes saved on my computer from almost every culture. Some of the foods not normally found in a cookbook include: African, Australian, Brazilian, Creol, Cuban, Czech, Korean, Polish, Russian, Swedish, and Thai dishes. I have recipes for canning and freezing; Crock-Pot, Dutch oven, and medieval cooking; pickle, cheese, sauerkraut, and sausage making; and smoking for both jerky and vegetables. In the past, I thought this was normal on a diet because saving recipes let me think about food instead of my hunger. Now I know better.

I can also testify that since I went on the RMR diet, I have not looked up a single recipe on the Internet. It has kept me from being in starvation mode, and I didn't even know it.

Starvation mode can cause your body to "break down proteins from your muscle tissue to use as fuel."[10] In many diet books, this is called "lean body mass." These sources leave people with the idea that lean body mass refers only to muscles. Such is not the case. Lean body mass is everything in your body except fat, bones, teeth, toe and fingernails, and hair. Everything else is made of protein. Every cell in our bodies is made of protein. That includes your heart, kidneys, brain, and all the rest. That is why going into the starvation mode presents risks to these organs.

To illustrate, in the extreme, what the lack of sufficient protein will do to the body, picture one of those starving children in a "Feed the Children" ad on TV. First, they burned up all their carbohydrates, and then they burned up all their fat. Then the body started burning itself (or its lean body mass) up. In another extreme example of this process, many people freed from the Nazi death camps and Japanese prisoner of war camps during WWII did not survive. The damage done to their hearts and other lean body mass organs was too severe to ever be reversed, even when they were once again given food.

As serious as all this is, preventing this disaster is easy. Determine your RMR, and don't cut below it to less than half your BMR calorie intake. If necessary, increase your calorie intake by a hundred or so calories.

Everything covered so far should help you understand why the RMR diet is the easiest weight loss program to follow and the surest way to maintain your weight for the rest of your life. For me, it has been so easy in comparison to everything else I have done. Since I have tailored the plan to my own tastes, it matches who I am and what I eat. Finding my RMR and sticking to it has almost been like finding a bottle, opening it, and releasing a genie who has granted all my weight loss wishes.

What this diet is *not* is possibly more important than what it is. Almost every diet I have ever been on has had one major flaw: there were strict rules on what I could and could not eat, which ultimately caused me to go off the diet. I was born loving certain foods, and my life just isn't as worthwhile without them. Since the RMR diet is not a diet that requires a specific way of eating or outlines specific foods that must or must not be eaten, everyone can go on it with the expectation that their basic way of eating does not need to change too drastically. What a refreshing difference and an empowering philosophy that will help you to get on the diet and stay on it.

Consider, for instance, all those dos and do-nots most diets lay on us. For example, *Parade Magazine* once devoted an entire issue to the topic of losing weight. Here is some of the advice that issue included:

- choose the right diet; not every plan is right for every person
- fill up on fiber
- toss out all those naughty little goodies that might prove too tempting
- tell every one; sit your family down and tell them your goals
- find an affordable trainer
- have an apple a day

- eat only when you're hungry
- schedule your snacks (the night before was recommended)[11]

And so it went. None of the advice is necessarily wrong for a given person, but the overwhelming amount of advice is just one more example of how to complicate what can be a relatively simple and rewarding process.

The RMR diet is not about eating some special foods to activate special hormones. It is not about loading up on certain foods, such as protein, and prohibiting other foods, such as carbohydrates. Nor is it about, conversely, eating vegetables and fruit and limiting protein. It is definitely not about getting so hungry you could chew off one of your arms. Just the reverse is true. It is not an eating plan decided by someone else, no matter how much of an expert he or she may be in health or nutrition. Others can't do that because they have no idea what your lifestyle is like and what you like to eat. And it is definitely not one of those highly advertised weight loss plans where you send them hundreds of dollars and they send you meals that may or may not be to your liking, and may or may not satisfy you. With these plans you will surely put your fat back on once you stop sending them the money.

But the most personally satisfying aspect of the RMR diet is its flexibility—it is not a diet that has lists of proscribed meals you must eat each day. None of your favorite foods or ways of eating is prohibited—at any time. It is not a diet that allows you to snack on your favorite food only now and then. On this diet, the only restriction on what you eat is on the number of calories you consume, and even that is more than allowed on most other diets. Therefore, this diet will not tell you what to eat, when to eat, or how much to eat. That is totally up to you as an individual. The only restriction is not to exceed your RMR limit. What you do and how you do it is totally up to you.

Physiologically, this is not a diet on which you must exercise to prevent the loss of lean body mass, as most others are. Obviously, the more you do exercise, the more fat you will burn, but even that is totally up to you.

It is not a diet on which you will lose weight so fast you need plastic surgery to tighten loose skin. It is not a diet that will rob your body of needed nutrients, minerals, and vitamins—assuming, of course, that your current manner of eating is getting you those needed items now. I'm not even going to mention the food pyramid. Everybody knows to follow that in order to be eating well.

RMR is founded on such basic principles that it works for people at all stages of life. It works well and safely for everyone from the young to the aged. Those of advanced age have an especially hard time with many eating plans because as people age, their BMR decreases. The older we get, the more our metabolism decreases. The sad result of this is the amount of food that kept us vital, healthy, and thin at age twenty, will have started putting fat on us before we're forty. The older one gets, the faster this process happens.

A doctor recently told me this eating plan is also excellent for people who have a surgical procedure to restrict the amount of food the stomach can accept. (I guess I should at least name the doctor who told me this; his name is Fred, and he's my son.)

Smaller meals and frequent snacks are advised in such cases. However, if food intake is not controlled, eventually the stomach will start expanding, more food can be accepted, and weight loss stops. Getting on this diet and staying on it will assure the surgery achieves all of the desired results.

One of the things that makes this diet easier and ultimately more successful is that you do need not jump in and try to do everything at once. Since it really is about making your life better and more rewarding on all levels, you can start with those things you find easiest, or perhaps only tackle one or two things that have caused you the most difficulty in the past.

Once again, the RMR diet is for everyone in need of burning fat. Such things as current overweight or obese status, gender, age, and level of physical activity in no way influence the results that can be achieved. All of which is to say, once more, it is a diet you design specifically for you. In the end, you will be the one to decide what you eat, when you eat, how much you eat, and what you do to burn fat. The easy part is that you can keep doing most of what you already do. And control your RMR limit in the way that best suits you.

NOTES

1. Beil, Laura, "As if losing weight isn't hard enough, keeping it off is even harder," *The Seattle Times*, June 29, 2005, http://seattletimes.nwsource. com/html/health/2002350905_healthweightgain29.html?syndication=rss.
2. The description I found online was this: "RMR Diet is a powerful three-in-one program to help you manage your diet, weight, and exercise program.

Using your personal details and activity level, the program calculates the optimum energy requirements to meet your desired weight loss target. By recording food consumption selected from a comprehensive database of over 6000 food items you can visually monitor your energy and nutrient intake against daily targets. A second module allows you to record your weight and graph it against your projected target weight. In the third exercise module you record your activities selected from a supplied database. You can then graphically balance your energy input and expenditure." Shareup LLC, "RMR Diet" Shareup Downloads, http://www.shareup.net/Home-Education/Home-Inventory/RMR-Diet-review-19305.html.

3. Centers for Disease Control and Prevention, "U.S. Obesity Trends 1985-2007" *Department of Health and Human Services.* http://www.cdc.gov/nccdphp/dnpa/obesity/trend/maps/ (accessed Aug 21, 2008).
4. shannasmithbrugueras, "What is the best weight-reducing diet?" *Yahoo! Answers.* http://answers.yahoo.com/question/index?qid=1006020705528 (accessed Aug 21, 2008).
5. Another good calculator can be found at: bodybuilding.com/fun/calrmr.htm.
6. In fact, fasting can even increase our metabolic rate for a short time. One report shows it takes about one hundred hours of fasting before this metabolic rate comes back down. M. Elia, "Effect of starvation and very low calorie diets on protein-energy interrelationships in lean and obese subjects" United Nations University, http://www.unu.edu/unupress/food2/UID07E/uid07e11.htm.
7. manewell, "The Truth about 'Starvation Mode' " *About.com Health: Calorie Count*, http://www.calorie-count.com/forums/post/28742.html
8. Shiomi Ryuu, "How can crash diets affect mental well being?" *Yahoo! Answers.* http://answers.yahoo.com/question/index?qid=20061116130152AAuP4bP.
9. Bulik, Cynthia M., Ph.D, and Nadine Taylor, M.S., R.D., "The Physical and Psychological Effects of Dieting" *About.com Health*, http://womenshealth.about.com/od/fitnessandhealth/a/exrunawayeating_2.htm.
10. Ryuu, "How can crash diets affect mental well being?"
11. See *Parade*, January 13, 2008.

Tools

Calorie book → *the Calorie Counter Annette B Natow 2013 2007

Measuring cups & spoons

Scale

Journal

tape measure

2

Helps for the RMR Diet

At first, all you need is a good calorie book, a set of measuring cups and spoons, and a small scale to measure a few ounces of meat, cheese, and other items whose calorie count is listed by weight. You will need a journal, forms, or some other way to record your daily intake of food. A number of electronic devices can accomplish this function. The importance of using a tape measure will be discussed later. Of course, a scale to measure how many pounds you lose is also rewarding. The scale is also important at first because you may need to lower your RMR goal by a hundred calories or so if you're not burning as much fat as you want. Sometimes you might even gain a little weight. To begin with, don't worry too much about changes in your weight. Since you are designing your own plan, a few adjustments now and then only serve to prove that you are finding what works for you.

In addition to measuring spoons, cups, and scales, a couple of other things are recommended. Hardware-wise the use of a tape measure is almost a must. The truth is that what a tape measure shows about your waist, buttocks, legs, and arms can actually be the best indication of the real benefits you are achieving. While it may sound like a contradiction, sometimes when your scale seems to be stuck in one spot, by measuring the different parts of your body, you can discover you are still burning fat.

Also, a pedometer, which can be purchased fairly cheaply, will give you an idea of how many steps you take daily. This will help show you how much more energy you are using as you lose weight and walk more during a day.

More should be said about what is needed to get answers to questions, techniques, and solutions. Most important of all is a computer connected to the World Wide Web. Many web searches have already been included so far to illustrate how valuable this will be. Many more will come.

A good calorie counting book is a must, and any bookstore will offer you a number of choices. The one I use is *The Calorie Counter* by Annette B. Natow, Ph.D. and Jo-Ann Heslin, M.A., R.D. It was published by Pocket Books, first in 2003, and then in 2007.

It is especially useful because in addition to the regular items you would expect, Section Two of the book contains 161 pages of the various restaurant chains from A&W to Winchell's Donuts. When you must eat out, the calories consumed then can be calculated. This section also offers the following advice regarding eating out: "The larger portion you are served, and the more variety you are offered, the more likely you are to over-eat. Go easy on super-sizes and choose wisely at buffets."

The second type of book that is a must is a cooking-lite guide. Again, there are multiple choices from cooking old-fashioned recipes with fewer calories to gourmet meals. One I found interesting is *The Biggest Loser Cookbook,* published by Holtbrink Publishers in 2006. In addition to a variety of recipes, it includes some of the stories of people who lost the most weight on the NBC weight-loss reality show of the same name. Of course, if you're really into cooking, nothing rivals the Internet. By searching "recipes lite," you will find hundreds of recipes for virtually every type of food and from every region of the world.

And last, but not least, is this book. Keep it handy, and refer to it often. There is far more important information in it than can be assimilated in just one reading. It was designed to be used as a support tool throughout the process of remaking the way you eat in life, and getting the results you've always dreamed of.

COUNTING CALORIES IN REAL LIFE
Let me give one example of how I made a simple change that allowed me to eat one of my beloved higher calorie foods in a smaller amount and

still end up satisfied. We're talking about spaghetti here. I was taught to make spaghetti by our neighbor, when I was only fourteen years old. Her name was Della Compagni.

Instead of sticking with my old recipe, I made a few changes. In the past when I had cooked spaghetti and Italian sausage, I would heap my plate, and have no room or desire for anything else. By the time I had finished, I would usually be stuffed—and gaining weight. With the RMR diet in mind, I knew I wouldn't be able to continue like that? But would I have to give up spaghetti? Heaven forbid! Who cared if other diets banned pasta of all kinds.

I grabbed the calorie counter book and began calculating. Two ounces of uncooked spaghetti (about a cup cooked) contains around 200 calories depending on the brand. By keeping track of the caloric content of everything I put into my sauce, I was able to calculate that ½ a cup of it was close to 105 calories.

One valuable tip was that after I had frazzled the ground beef, I would fill the pan with hot water and then drain it. This got rid of all the grease. Another trick was that I'd limit the amount of olive oil for sautéing to two teaspoons, and keep the heat a little lower so as not to burn the vegetables such as garlic, onions, and mushrooms.

My new lunch contained the combined 305 calories of spaghetti, a small salad consisting of a cup and a half of red leaf lettuce (12 calories), half a cup of sliced cucumber (7 calories), one tablespoon chopped green onion (2 calories) and ten squirts of Wishbone Red Wine Salad Spritzers (10 calories). I also had half a cup of boiled green beans from my garden (22 calories). I prefer French bread with my spaghetti, rather than Italian, so one ounce of that (without butter) was an additional 75 calories. I had planned on finishing off my lunch with an apple, but by the time I'd eaten the 433 calories listed above, I found I was fully satisfied.

All this detail and background is to illustrate some vital points about any meal, whether it be home cooked or at a restaurant. The first is that no matter what your favorite foods are, with a little care and combination with other foods, you can eat, enjoy, and be satisfied while still staying within your RMR limits.

The second is that by calculating the caloric content of everything in a combination dish, such as the spaghetti sauce, then measuring the total volume or weight, we can obtain a fairly accurate count of how many calories are in a given portion. While this may be a little complicated the first time the dish is prepared, once that's done you will know how much you can have from then on.

Obviously, by buying bottles of spaghetti sauce from Prego or Ragu, all you have to do is check the nutritional info on the label. The same goes for any other commercially prepared food.

Another thing to remember is that, at best, calorie counting is nothing but close approximations. Different calorie books will sometimes list slightly different calories for the same foods. Some of the calorie amounts I listed came from the packages for that food, and different brands will vary. One example is the spaghetti I referred to; it was actually fettucini. I also have some thin spaghetti, which has 110 calories for the same amount of pasta.

As long as you stay reasonably confident that you are not exceeding your RMR limit, exactly how many calories you consume is neither significant nor possible to calculate. For example, when I'm looking something up, I always round it off to the nearest five calories. Twenty-two calories gets listed as twenty, and twenty-three calories gets listed as twenty-five. When adding all my calories up, it's a lot easier, and in the long run it averages out.

While I was specific in my calculations of the green beans and salad, for instance, in practice I only estimate what that would be, since they are such low-calorie foods, and being off by ten or twenty calories one way or another is not a tragedy. Of course, such estimations are based on considerable experience of having looked up and recorded that food in the past. It's nice to know the longer one stays on this eating plan, the easier it gets as our knowledge about the caloric values of what we eat grows.

CHOOSING THE RIGHT FOODS

In choosing day by day what food you will eat, it is very wise to make sure that foods you find acceptable will also help you to maintain proper nutrition. Once that's said, the store's the limit. You will not have to plan your meals out a week in advance, unless that's the sort of thing you like doing. You can even make up your mind what you want to eat for a given meal as late as when you start preparing it.

One useful question for me is "Let's see, what am I in the mood for?" One can't plan that out in advance, and answering it each time definitely goes a long way toward making what one eats far more satisfying. This goes for both meals and snacks. Of course, it is also necessary sometimes to settle for what is on hand or left over in the icebox.

Thus, what one eats has only three important tests: Will it be satisfying? How will I keep track of the caloric content of this food? Overall, is it meeting my nutritional needs? This works well. Once you decide what to eat, it works well to determine the caloric content of the items to be eaten, and what quantity will be eaten to stay within your RMR limit.

That's where the calorie book, measuring spoons, and portion scale come in handy. Before you ever sit down to eat, you can know you will be eating something enjoyable, and just how much of it you will be eating. Another step is to log the meal into a calorie sheet, electronic device, or journal before you eat it. It is easier to resist that little extra something if resisting it also means you are not going to have to change your record.

While a minimum of two meals per day are recommended, research has proven breakfast is the most important meal of the day. It cannot be overemphasized that no matter what one's lifestyle is, this eating plan will be more effective if it includes breakfast.

What's for breakfast? Shall we have bagels and cream cheese or a couple of fried eggs, toast, and jam? Believe it or not there was actually a study done on this very question. I found an article titled "Breakfast: Bagel vs. Eggs" that outlined a study showing people who ate the eggs not only ate less for lunch and supper but lost more weight. According to the study, "overweight and obese women who consumed a breakfast of two eggs a day (for five days a week or more) for 8 weeks, as part of a low-fat diet with a 1,000 calorie deficit: lost 65 percent more weight, had 83 percent greater reduction in waist circumference, reported greater improvement in energy levels than their dieting counterparts who consumed a bagel breakfast of the same calories."[1]

I tried it myself, but I ate only one egg, an ounce or two of smoked salmon or extra-lean ham, and a slice of bread without any butter. I was a little mystified to discover that, for me, this kind of breakfast works. I began to be less hungry throughout the day. To this day I do not understand how this paltry breakfast can cut down so much on my desire for food, especially in the morning until it's time to eat lunch. I often have to remind myself I should have a snack before lunch.

The message here is not that bagels are bad, but that eggs in the morning have salutary effects. As long as you counts your calories, bagels during any other part of the day seem to be no problem.

There is a lot more latitude when it comes to eating lunch, or supper, or both. While breakfast is a must, beyond that your lifestyle will determine what you choose, or are able to get, at any given meal.

If you have a job, you may have to eat on the run for lunch. According to one article I read, this can be dangerous.

> When we eat outside the home, "portions go up and nutrition goes down," says Kelly D. Brownell, director of The Rudd Center for Food Policy and Obesity at Yale University. . . .
>
> A whopping 75 percent of office workers eat at their desks two or three times a week, according to the American Dietetic Association. If you do, prepare something healthy and satisfying in advance. Bring in nutritious snacks as well, for energy to stave off hunger. Otherwise, it's too easy to help yourself to whatever is available. A study at the University of Illinois at Urbana-Champaign found that secretaries whose candy dishes were close at hand ate more than twice as many chocolates as those whose dishes were six feet away. . . .[2]

For about four years now I've been substitute teaching for three days a week. When I first learned about the RMR eating process, this problem of what to eat while away from home arose for me. How would I snack, and what would I eat for lunch? I found that frozen, prepackaged, microwaveable meals such as Stouffer's Lean Cuisine roasted garlic chicken (180 calories) not only worked fine but were enjoyable as well. I'd heat them up in the teacher's lounge during lunch.

I had to stay especially conscious of the calories in some of these "diet" frozen meals. When I started looking at them I began to wonder how some of them could consider so many calories "eating lite." Plus, I had to experiment a bit to discover which ones I liked and which had more of the consistency of wet cardboard than any food I enjoyed.

In the little carrying case I take to school with me, I also began carrying things like baby carrots in a baggie, a small banana, a small apple, or even a baggie of feta cheese. I could easily snack on such items, consuming all or part of them in the five minute break between classes. I also carried small salt and pepper shakers. Some things just aren't palatable without salt. Of course, a person with high blood pressure does not have this luxury.

Lunch at home may or not be your main meal of the day. For me, on those days I'm not teaching, lunch is my main meal. Again, the most important questions for anyone are, "What sounds good today, and how much of it can I eat?"

Whatever type of food you choose for meals, good nutrition is especially important because of the lowered total calories you are consuming each day. Some things you used to eat may not be part of your new eating plans, and even those foods you still eat might now be eaten in smaller portions and may no longer provide the nutrition they did before the RMR diet.

It is important to become familiar with the food pyramid and follow its general guidelines so that you eat the right amounts of the right variety of foods. You should also understand that the pyramid is merely an approximation of what individuals need, and you should recognize that different people will have different pyramid needs. When going online one source that comes up is MyPyramid.gov. It lists twelve different models for different circumstances. People with diabetes have one, and elderly people have another.

One pyramid gives the following suggestions for appropriate servings:

Fats, oils and sweets—use sparingly
Dairy—2 to 3 servings
Proteins—2 to 3 servings
Fruits—2 to 4 servings
Vegetables—3 to 5 servings
Breads and grains—6 to 11 servings.

This same source also gives examples of what constitutes a serving for each food group:

Bread, grains, cereal and pasta—1 slice of bread; ½ cup of rice, cooked cereal or pasta; 1 cup of ready-to-eat cereal; 1 flat tortilla.
Vegetables—1 cup of raw leafy vegetables; ½ cup of other vegetables, cooked or raw; ¾ cups vegetable juice.
Fruits—1 medium apple, orange, or banana; ½ cup of chopped, cooked, or canned fruit; ¾ cups 100 percent fruit juice.
Beans, eggs, lean meat and fish—1 egg, 2 tablespoons of peanut butter, ½ cup of cooked beans, and ¼ cup of nuts.

They don't specify what a serving of meat includes because you can have more of one, such as fish, and less of another, such as steak. However they do advise, "Choose lean meat, fish, and dry beans and peas often because these are the lowest in fat. Remove skin from poultry and trim away visible fat on meat. Avoid frying these foods."

There are two things I'd like to mention here. The first is that while you can search the Internet for the many serving recommendations, it is generally accepted that the package nutrition information on most items will usually give what is considered as one serving. If the amount of that item that is to be served does not match the label, it can always be looked up in the calorie book.

Second, frying foods (including eggs) can fit into the food pyramid if vegetable sprays are used to lubricate the frying pan, or if the amount of oil called for in the recipe is greatly reduced. Vegetable sprays have zero calories and zero fat. If the recipe calls for frying with or adding butter, the margarine Brown and Brummel® is much lower in calories than most other margarines, and far lower in calories than butter.

Further information about how many servings we should have is stated in the above article when it quotes what the Department of Agriculture says about these recommendations: "The advised numbers of servings from each group varies depending on how many calories you take in each day. This, in turn, depends on your activity level, body size, gender, age, and stage of life."[3]

Once all this is considered, the truth of the statement that the food pyramid is a guideline can be better understood. It is just a guideline. One need not worry that every meal or every day must strictly conform to what is indicated there. As long as the required ingredients are consumed over the course of the week, that will be just fine.

One caution here is that most of those fats you do get should be of the healthy variety, and even then, it pays to reduce fat intake. Jay S. Cohen, MD, says:

> The lesson is that Atkins, who said "All fats are good," was wrong. Good fats are good, and bad fats are bad. Americans consume large quantities of bad fats—saturated fats and hydrogenated oils—that elevate cholesterol levels and cause cardiovascular disease. Indeed, every society that has adopted western dietary habits has suffered major increases in heart attacks and strokes. People from diet-healthy societies who come here and adopt our ways of eating get all of our diseases.
>
> Advocates of low-fat diets with moderate amounts of protein and high-quality complex carbohydrates have plenty of evidence supporting their perspective. Studies repeatedly show that when people stick with low-fat diets, incidences of coronary disorders, heart attacks, and cardiac deaths plummet.[4]

Therefore, to plan your meals around the pyramid, breakfast, might be high on dairy, protein, and cereals, while lunch would fill in with vegetables, fruit, pasta, and a few nuts. Different snacks throughout the day could supplement with smaller portions as required.

Lunch and supper (whether you eat one or both) can be eaten at any time one chooses. One guideline however is that the body works best if meals are eaten roughly at the same time every day.

Whether or not a particular meal is high or low in calories is not important either, as long as the caloric RMR limit for the day is not exceeded. Depending on what one chooses for your own eating plan, one meal can be high in calories as long as other meals and snacks are lower. More important is the quantities one eats at mealtimes. By reducing how much volume of food you eat, your body will soon adjust to that smaller volume.

SUBSTITUTIONS

Following are some examples of how the different choices one makes can easily contribute to that goal. All calories listed are for the same quantities (except where specified), but are simply close approximations since different calorie books frequently give slightly different values for the same food.

SUBSTITUTIONS				
Item	Serving size	Calories	Substitute	Calories
Regular Butter	1 T	100	Brown & Brummel® margarine	45
Bacon cooked	1 oz	162	Ham roasted	59
Chuck blade roast	3 oz	215	Chuck arm roast	178
T-bone Steak	3 oz	182	Sirloin steak	162
Regular hamburger	3 oz	244	Extra lean	213
Tuna in oil	2 oz	160	Tuna in water	60
Bagel (Sarah Lee®)	1	190	Biscuit (Wonder®)	80
Cooked rice	4 oz	111	Boiled potato	99

SUBSTITUTIONS				
Item	Serving size	Calories	Substitute	Calories
Cooked corn	1 cup	166	Green beans	44
Banana	1	120	Blueberries (1 cup)	81
Apple	1 cup	65	Watermelon	51
Sugar (white)	1 cup	773	Sugar substitutes	0

While hundreds of such examples could be listed, the above should demonstrate that there are many, many different substitutions that can be made to keep you well within your RMR limit. But in choosing any one type of food over another, what you really enjoy is equally as important as caloric content. For example, what meat lover wouldn't choose prime rib over pot roast? Even if it meant eating a little less.

Much of the preceding is of more value to those with the time, energy, and luxury of cooking. In our sometimes hectic lifestyles, we often settle for packaged, canned, or frozen food, for part, if not all, of the meal.

Anyone old enough to read this book is probably already familiar with the great number of such items from the store shelves, the cooler section, or the freezer section. The variety of pre-prepared and pre-packaged foods is so wide and the choices so varied, they will suffice for almost any type of eating plan. This variety also means something can be found that fits almost everyone's likes and dislikes.

However, when it comes to nutrition, certain guidelines apply with pre-packaged foods as well. Always read the nutrition information labels. First is the serving size. Will it be large enough to be adequate for the purpose intended, or will a smaller amount have to be used? Second is the calories. Will one or two servings fit generally into the day's RMR limit? Third is the fat content. What is the fat content of the items and what percent of the total calories come from fat? Whatever level of BMR one is on, the food pyramid puts fat at the very top and has the comment, "use sparingly."

While such things as the sugar in candy is discouraged because it provides no nutrition in the calories consumed, the overconsumption of fats carries considerable health risks. Over time, clogged arteries, heart attacks, and strokes have all been linked to excessive consumption of these fats.

We also need to be on the lookout when we read "no trans fats" on a label. This often means more acceptable forms of fat, such as olive oil or canola oil are being used. Whether eating trans fats such as butter, or unsaturated (trans fat free) items such as olive and canola oil, any excess brings on the problems listed. Unsaturated fats just take a little more of the fats to cause them and brings the problems on a little slower.

The key to all of this is comparison shopping—not comparing price, but comparing nutrition values. Nor should one simply grab what has always been used and enjoyed. By looking around at similar items, it is usually possible to find a different brand that is equally enjoyable and contains far fewer calories.

True, as often as not, the substitute might be lacking a certain appeal. But by experimenting with items not previously tried, one can definitely improve the types and variety of foods eaten. All of this makes this life-long metabolic eating plan far more enjoyable and significantly healthier.

SNACKS

Now that main meals have been covered, when it comes to snacks all the general rules of calories and nutrition still apply, but there are two main differences. The first is that, when possible, snacks should really be savored and enjoyed. Second, they should also help satisfy feelings of increased appetite. For these reasons, snacks are equally if not more important than meals themselves in the nutritional value they bring to an eating plan.

Some studies suggest a minimum of three snacks in addition to your regular meals, but more are recommended. Ten snacks a day? That's right. One of them might be five green olives (25 calories). Another might be a dill pickle (10 calories). Or even a sandwich with one slice of Sarah Lee's® 100 percent multi-grain bread (45 calories), half a dill pickle (5 calories) and a tablespoon of ketchup (8 calories) if you want a little more to munch on.

There are a couple of suggestions to help make snacks what they need to be. The first is to beware of unconscious snacking. Don't glom on to something from the counter every time you pass by and throw it into your "big bazoo." Choose your snacks carefully and stay conscious of the fact that you are eating them. Let the body zip in that feeling of satisfaction.

The following is only a small list of the snacks available. These few are listed to show that in every food category there are numerous possibilities, and to spark some ideas for those who are not used to thinking of snacks as part of a fat-burning process or a nutritional diet.

Low-calorie Healthy Snacks		
Item	Serving size	Calories
DAIRY (high in protein and calcium)		
Non-fat milk	1 cup	80
Non-fat sour cream	2 T	20
Yogurt (Dannon® Lite & Fit)	1 cup	80
NUTS (protein-rich)		
Almonds	⅛ cup	103
Cashews (dry roasted)	9 nuts	80
Peanuts (dry roasted)	15 nuts	85
Sunflower seeds	⅛ cup	100
PROTEIN		
Egg (boiled)	1 egg	85
Beef jerky	2 pieces	80
Thinly sliced ham, turkey, or roast beef (Buddig™)	5 slices	40
Tuna (in water)	½ can	60
CHEESE (protein-rich, but usually high in fat)		
Cheddar	1 oz	110
Cheddar (low fat)	1 oz	49
Colby	1 oz	110
Cottage (low fat)	½ cup	80
Feta (goat cheese)	1 oz	75
Swiss (light)	1 oz	80
FRUITS (Fresh fruits are generally lower in calories than fruit juices.)		

Low-calorie Healthy Snacks		
Item	Serving size	Calories
Apple	1 large	110
Banana	1 extra small	72
Cantaloupe	1 half	94
Cantaloupe	1 cup	57
Cranberries (fresh chopped)	1 cup	54
Cranberry juice low calorie cocktail (as an exception to the above)	6 oz	33
Orange (navel)	one	65
Orange (valencia)	one	59
Peach	one	50
Plum	one	36
Prunes	¼ cup	110
Raisins	¼ cup	130
Watermelon	1 cup	50
Vegetables (High water content makes fruits and vegetables very filling for relatively few calories.)		
Broccoli (raw)	1 cup	20
Carrot (raw)	1 baby	6
Carrot (raw)	1 regular size	31
Cauliflower (raw or cooked)	1 cup	28
Olive (green)	one extra large	5
Olive (Greek)	one	10
Olive (black)	one	5
Dill pickle	one	12
Sweet pickle	one	41
Sweet gherkin	one	20
Carbohydrates		

LOW-CALORIE HEALTHY SNACKS		
Item	Serving size	Calories
Bread (Sarah Lee® multigrain)	1 slice	45
Pasta (various)	½ cup	80–100
Pretzels	1 oz	108
Rice (brown, grained, cooked)	½ cup	108
Rice (white, cooked)	½ cup	103
Sushi (California roll)	1 piece	28
Tortilla chips	3 chips	35
Baked potato	one half	110

Every supermarket contains dozens of so-called health food snacks. Health food stores contain even more. As long as wise comparison shopping is done, some of these will certainly contribute to the enjoyment, nutrition, and workability of the RMR plan.[5]

It's important to mention, however, that many snacks need not be solitary items we just grab and eat. For example, one package of green olive chip dip mixed into a cup of fat-free sour cream only comes to about twenty-five calories per two tablespoon servings. If you took three tortilla chips and dipped them in the mix, this would come to only around fifty calories total.

Half of a five-ounce baked potato (without the skin) and two tablespoons of fat-free sour cream is only about ninety calories. By using non-fat yogurt instead of cream, even that can be cut. But let's not forget leftovers. Some cooked veggies such as cauliflower, broccoli, or asparagus that weren't eaten earlier might just fill the bill. Even a little of that high calorie stuff you enjoyed so much for lunch is not out of line taken in snack-sized portions.

A close look at what has just been said can illustrate some important things. One is that the particular brand names I mentioned all have a lower calorie content than most similar items on the store shelf. Choosing lower-calorie brands not only helps keep you within your RMR, but it can also allow you to eat more while doing it.

It is not necessary to have specific snacks lined up for a given day. What you think early in the day might be a grand snack later can easily change depending on a lot of factors. What seems to work far better, especially when it comes to being satisfied, is to wait until it's time to snack and then choose one that will be most enjoyable right then.

Thus, having a large variety of different snacks available to choose from is a sound plan. The only caution here is not to have several of them right there in sight if just seeing them can cause you to want them. Keeping them in the cupboard and the icebox works best.

Snacks are not things that should just happen. By staying conscious of our caloric intake for the day up to that time, as well as how we feel or what we want, we can make snacks work for us instead of against us.

So far, candy has not been mentioned as a snack. Properly used, candy is perfectly acceptable as long as you keep your total calorie intake within your RMR limit for the day. The problem is that some of us are addicted to chocolate, or other favorite candies. For example, to me there are only two flavors of ice cream. Chocolate, and everything else. The causes of this addiction can range from acquiring it as a child in the form of a reward from our parents, to emotionally eating it when we're unhappy or something upsets us. "Eating chocolate releases chemicals similar to those released when you fall in love; to overcome addiction you need to understand the cause behind it. . . . Set a daily quota for chocolate, come what may, do not exceed; view it as a form of indulgence, a prize for yourself."[6]

However, there are other tips on controlling the addiction instead of letting it control us. One is not having the food in plain sight. As reported earlier, secretaries whose candy dishes were close at hand ate twice as much as those whose dishes were six feet away. Sometimes it's hard to believe that such a little change could have such valuable results.

Another change is not buying large amounts of candy at any one time. Few of us are so addicted that we'll blow a whole day if we have to go to the store to get more, once we've eaten the little we have on hand.

Then there is the matter of substitution. Many people, me included, find they don't really need a Hershey's® bar if they can have something sweet that contains chocolate. Just two examples from one producer are Quaker® Chewy Chocolate Chip Granola bars (100 calories each); and Quaker® Mini Delights Chocolatey Drizzle (90 calories per package).

Then there is the old admonition, "Moderation in all things." It is both possible and satisfying to only eat a small part of any given delight.

Half a Hershey's® bar only contains half the calories. One quarter of one contains even less. One or two squares per day will not ruin any eating plan. But perhaps the best news of all is that now we can buy sugar-free chocolate. There are hardly any calories in that at all, and it is just as satisfying as the other kind.

NOTES

1. Jillon S. Vander Wal, PhD; Jorene M. Marth, MA, RD; Pramod Khosla, PhD, K-L; Catherine Jen, PhD; and Nikhil V. Dhurandhar, PhD, FACN. "Short-Term Effect of Eggs on Satiety in Overweight and Obese Subjects," *Journal of the American College of Nutrution* 24, no. 6 (2005):510–515, (as quoted in Foster, J., "Breakfast: Bagel vs. Eggs," Diet-Blog, http://www.diet-blog.com/archives/2007/05/10/breakfast_bagel_vs_eggs.php).
2. Schnurnberger, Lynn, "Healthy Ways to Eat on the Run," *Parade*, March 30, 2008, 31.
3. Lifeclinic: Health Management Systems, "Food Guide Pyramid," Lifeclinic Intl, http://www.lifeclinic.com/focus/nutrition/food-pyramid.asp
4. Jay S. Cohen M.D., "Low Fat Diets Don't Work? Don't Believe It! Headlines Misrepresent Studies," MedicationSense, http://www.medicationsense.com/articles/jan_apr_06/low_fat_diet_021606.html.
5. You can find a good list of healthy snacks online, compiled by the University of Nebraska. (Boeckner, Linda S. and Karen L. Schledewitz, "It's Snack Time," University of Nebraska, http://elkhorn.unl.edu/epublic/live/g1033/build/).
6. stargazing, "Help, how do I overcome a chocolate addiction?" *Yahoo! Answers*, http://answers.yahoo.com/question/index?qid=1006012908788 (accessed Aug 26, 2008).

3

Controlled Weight Loss

Fat burning is not a constant. Any dietician (or anyone else for that matter) who tells us that we can expect to burn a given amount of fat every week does not have a firm grasp on reality. Sometimes our body holds onto more water than at other times. If we have an infection, the body might well turn up its heat (what calories produce when they're burned) to fight that infection. If we are cold, we will burn more calories, and the reverse is true if we're hot.

One thing is certain, in the short run, any fat our scales show was gone may only be an illusion. One of the reasons it is an illusion is that the first few pounds may well be just a drop in the amount of water you were retaining. I have found that I can pretty well trust a weight change that has persisted over a month's time.

It's not that seeing a drop of two pounds over a week or two week period is not significant. As has already been mentioned, losing such an amount means your RMR limit is fairly accurate, your calorie counting is fairly accurate, and you are eating the right amount of food at the right times of the day. All of these are good things, but the biggest benefit is, that it makes us happy to see our weight going down. While one week without a loss doesn't plunge us into despair, two weeks can definitely make us cranky.

If, early on, you are not getting the results desired, discovering the problems should be easy. Begin reducing your total intake by a hundred calories per day until an acceptable weight loss is being accomplished. One caution here—look at any diet book authored by a doctor or a nutritionist

29

and you will see that one to two pounds per week is the maximum you should lose. In fact, anything more than a pound a week can have health risks.[1]

However, if you show no weight loss for more than about two weeks, it is important to search the records of daily consumption you have kept. A couple of things need to be determined. First, if this is the first time this has happened, it will probably change soon. If it goes on, a records check can help you determine if you are really eating what you should, or if you are, eating more than you thought you were.

THE PLATEAU SYNDROME

If you really seem to be stalled, you might be stuck in what is called the Plateau Syndrome. This can be extremely serious with regards to staying on a diet. One cause of this syndrome is the starvation mode, which has already been covered. But another problem is that if you do not know what is happening to you, your natural tendency is to believe the diet is no longer working. In my own case in the past, this was a real diet buster and caused me to regain all the weight I'd lost, and at times, to gain even more.

By searching "Diet Plateau Syndrome" on the Internet, as usual, there are hundreds of sources available. I found one article particularly useful.

> The most important thing to remember is that this is a completely normal experience for many dieters. The key to success is not allowing yourself to become discouraged! . . .
>
> A plateau may occur because your body simply wants a "rest" to cope with your calorie reduction; your calorie intake equals your calorie expenditure; [or] you have reduced your calorie intake too low. . . . The closer you get to your goal weight, the slower the weight tends to come off. . . . There are weeks when you simply retain fluids and weigh a pound or two more than you did the week before.[2]

If the plateau goes on for enough time that you know something has to be done, this article also covers that.

> Avoid weighing yourself too frequently—once a week is enough. . . . Weigh yourself once a week at the same time, after the same routine, and on the same scales. . . . Sometimes a better way to judge whether you are slimming down and changing body shape is just by monitoring how your clothes feel. . . .
>
> Go back to keeping your food diary religiously. By tracking what

you eat, you may discover that you're actually consuming a good deal more calories than you'd imagined. . . .

Start exercising! To lose weight you need to burn more calories than you consume. . . .

Step up your exercise level [if you are already exercising]. . . .

Drink plenty of water! Water helps speed up the metabolism. . . .

Don't starve yourself—this will have the opposite effect! . . . Ideally, eat something such as a piece of fruit every 3 hours (women) or 5 hours (men). . . .

Be determined! Focus on your successes to date and remember that weight loss is simply about creating an energy deficit.

Another article confirmed the advice to drink more water and specified how much water to drink. It advised at least two liters (approximately two quarts), then went on to say, "You may consume up to 3 ounces of the following protein foods 5 times a day: beef, pork, chicken, turkey, lamb, fish, eggs, low-fat cheese, cottage cheese, plain yogurt or artificially sweetened, peanut butter, beans, and legumes." It also emphasized exercise and advised trying to get at least thirty minutes per day."[3]

Some of the people who used this advice wrote testimonials on the site about how well it worked for them. But a couple complained that all that protein caused them constipation and that they had to take something to relieve that.

Another article gave more information on the reason water is so important.

Water is essential for your body to metabolize stored fat into energy—so much so, that your body's metabolism can be slowed by relatively mild levels of dehydration. And the slower your metabolism, the slower your weight loss (and the greater your fatigue), until eventually your weight loss just crawls to a halt, and you hit the dreaded diet plateau.

Water is a natural appetite suppressant. In the hypothalamus, a region in your brain that controls appetites and cravings, the control centers for hunger and thirst are located next to each other. . . . Chronic mild dehydration can confuse these control mechanisms, leading to feelings of hunger, rather than thirst.[4]

The article "How to Break Out of a Weight Loss Plateau" recommends a minimum of 1200 calories per day for women and 1500 per day for men. Regarding more protein, the author advises, "You may try to break a plateau by decreasing the percentage of carbohydrates and increasing the percentage of protein that you intake each day."[5]

My own experiences on this subject might prove useful. The amazing thing about the RMR diet was that I did not even experience a plateau until I'd lost fifty-three pounds. Since I still weighed 195 at the time, I knew I was close enough to my goal that I was not going to let this stop me.

I started drinking a little more liquid, stayed on my diet, and waited. Two weeks went by, and then a third with no weight loss. Obviously, the plateau ended, but the most important part of it was that while my weight was stalled I was still burning fat. The proof? My belt needed two more notches to get tight and my pants size went from 40 to 38! Go figure.

THE SNACK ATTACK

Another diet buster is the snack attack. How important snacks are to the RMR diet has already been covered. There are three basic rules regarding snacks to keep them from becoming diet busters. First, we must snack reasonably frequently. Second, our snacks are to be used to stave off hunger pangs. Third, when possible, snacks should be something we enjoy at that particular time.

What has not been covered is how snacks pervade what most people eat, how the food industry promotes them, and how they can be one of the causes of our climbing obesity rates.

Because all of us have such a history of snacking, we need understand how not controlling our snack attacks can ruin our diet. And, equally important, we need to fully understand the tremendous difference between our past snacking and what we need to do now. Finally, we must do everything we can to utilize the type of snacks we need, while controlling those that bust our diets.

As with everything else in this book, unless snacking is not a problem for you, controlling your snacks should not be attempted all at once. Usually, the great amount of willpower and resolve we have at the start of a project will fade over time. More effective is a steely determination that we will stick with something until we achieve exactly what we want.

Here are some of the things that motivate almost everyone to snack. We just grab something because it was there. Often, we're not even conscious we've done it. Or perhaps it was something we became accustomed to doing at certain times of the day or in certain circumstances. Perhaps we get a chocolate donut on the way to work. Or we have a package of Twinkies during our break. Or we get a package of Doritos when we go into the gas station to pay for our gas.

This brings up the tremendous snack food industry. What most of them call snacks hardly fit into our RMR diet, unless we eat only a portion of them. Just how pervasive that industry is can be discovered by going online and entering either "diet snacking" or just "snacks." Surprisingly, you'll find a large percentage of the entries by producers of one type of food or another vying for your money.

You'll also be amazed at the number of companies who are only too happy to help you. Many have reduced calories, or put out smaller portions.

Another motivation to snack is that certain snacks simply call to us. We may have enjoyed them since childhood. There are few among us who would include items like celery, carrots, broccoli, or a hunk of cabbage on that list. One thing is almost certain, however, we eat far too many of the unhealthy items because we think of them often.

Then there are the things we have become accustomed to getting when we feel hungry. These are generally sweets for women or salty foods for men. That means a woman may go for a candy bar, a piece of pie or cake, or graham crackers. A man gets a hunk of cheese, a package of potato chips, or a package of salted nuts. Maybe all three at once. Naturally, this sex difference is not an iron-clad certainty. Some women like salty as well, and some men go for sweet.

Perhaps the most dangerous snacks are what I call shared snacks. They generally begin with something like, "Honey, would you like some ice cream?" Another type of shared snack is when you're out with a friend: "Let's get a pizza," or a banana split, or whatever. Even if you are not the one suggesting it, this type of snack is hard to refuse. First, because you want that too, and second, because you don't want to appear to be a "dork" in front of your friend. I won't even mention the overweight friend who may be jealous of the weight you are losing and who may even want to sabotage you.

Snacks also depend on our time off life. Whether you're a pre-teen, a teenager, a young adult, a middle-aged adult, or nearly senile, you are in a group that has their favorite snacks. This is not always bad. In fact, certain ages really do better when snacking. Young children's tiny stomachs can hold only small portions of food at one time. Older adults who are less active and who burn fewer calories also may feel more comfortable eating smaller meals more frequently.[6]

This same article then explains some reasons to promote snacks including "binge control," "extra energy," and "nutrients." It continues, "plan [snacks] with variety, moderation, and balance in mind."

The types of foods this article recommends for snacks are "whole grains, fruits and vegetables, nuts and seeds and low-fat dairy products." Then they also provide a chart of snacks by calorie content.

10 calories	1 large stalk of celery
25–30 calories	1 cup raw vegetables 6 medium baby carrots
60 calories	2 cups air-popped or light popcorn 1 cup of cantaloupe or grapes 1 small can of vegetable juice
100 calories	1 cup sliced bananas and fresh raspberries 2 domino-sized slices low-fat Colby or cheddar cheese 1 fat-free chocolate pudding cup
150 calories	½ cup frozen, low-fat yogurt topped with ½ cup blueberries 1 cup sliced apples with 1 tablespoon smooth peanut butter 4 slices whole-grain crispbread crackers (a wafer-thin cracker)
200 calories	¼ cup dry roasted soy nuts (calories vary by brand) ⅓ cup granola 1 cup low-fat cottage cheese topped with ½ cup sliced fresh peaches

Another article gives useful info on how to prepare your own one hundred calorie or fewer snacks.

You may have seen those expensive little prepackaged snacks that guarantee to only have 100 calories. Don't spend your hard-earned cash on them! You can make your own at home in just a few minutes. . . .

Take a look on the label of your favorite snack first. How much is one serving?

Next, how many calories are in one serving?

Now, to figure out how much of your treat you will need to make a 100-calorie snack sack, take the amount of calories and divide it by 100. Then, divide the serving amount by the number you come up with. For example, if your treat is candy and a serving is one cup at 350 calories, you would take 350 and divide it by 100. That would come out to 3.5. So, you would divide that 1 cup serving by 3.5. That would give you about one-third of a cup of candy for your snack pack.

Finally measure the snack and put it in [a] baggie.[7]

If you divide the total calories by two hundred, you can come up with a fifty-calorie serving. Naturally, if your favorite snack comes in a large container, you will end up with a number of baggies.

The trick here is to make sure you limit yourself as to how many of these you will have in a day. To obtain the full value of snacking for the RMR diet, you need to have a number of different items for snacks, not just one type of snack that you eat a number of times throughout the day.

FOOD DIARY

Switching gears, a way to record your daily calorie intake was also mentioned as a must. One thing I found useful was a three-ring binder I could put a number of items in, such as daily calorie and food sheets, lined paper for making notes, my diet plan, and articles I came across that I found useful.

However, whether you're doing it electronically, on paper forms, or in a diary or a journal, much more than your daily calories and foods needs to be recorded. You need to record the weight you are losing, and the date you first weighed that.

If you've achieved something you're proud of or something that gave you pleasure, that needs to go in as well. Conversely, if you had a problem of some kind, record that, and how you solved it. You need to jot down any little tricks or other aids you've found to make the whole process easier. The RMR eating plan is a lifelong endeavor that will improve your life on every level. As such, after some time has passed, you might forget what your successes and failures were, what made you happy, and what irritated you. Recording it as you go lets you review those feelings from time to time and helps to keep you balanced.

One extremely important thing to keep in a journal is what was going on when you ate something you shouldn't have or overate at a meal. Were you angry? Were you upset at someone or something? Were you sad? Were you excited? All these things can and do contribute to overeating. By being aware and logging them into the journal, you can begin to recognize them and keep them from ruining the diet.

There are some things I've learned that you may find useful. One is to record your calories as soon as you eat them. Too many times, I vowed I would remember and log in my calories the next time I was near the sheets I keep in my journal. You already know the rest of the story. Either I would forget that I had eaten something, or I would not be able to remember just how much of it I ate.

I'm sure you've heard the old saying: "Live and learn." Well, at my age it's: "Live and learn, and wake up in the morning and forget it all." That's why I carry one of those small, spiral-bound notebooks with me to log down anything I eat, think of, or experience when I can't put it on my record sheet or in my journal immediately.

One of the big advantages I find in logging calories right away is that I can add up what I've eaten so far in a given day to help me gauge what to do for the rest of the day to keep within my RMR limit. Now comes one of the most important rules for making all your recorded information most valuable to you—review it often!

PORTION CREEP

As time goes by, you will become familiar with both the approximate amount and calorie content of various foods. Some you will have served often enough that you know enough to just log everything into the journal without measuring it or looking it up. And finally, you might become so familiar with the food you eat, that you will just know what to eat, how much to eat, and when to eat it.

Since the RMR diet is a lifelong change in eating, you can't go on for the rest of your life measuring, looking up calorie content, and logging it down. But don't rush this process! If you do, you are in danger of encountering what is called "portion creep," which will destroy all you have done. Portion creep is rampant both in our society, and in individuals who have become overweight or obese.

The great danger here is pretty well described in the name. It creeps up on you, slowly, over time, and you're probably not even aware it is happening. Your body adjusts to the slowly increasing portions until you soon begin to feel that this amount is normal.

When we stop measuring and counting, we have only one defense against this insidious condition—our scales. The moment you stop losing weight (and you're not just on a plateau) or when you begin to add even a couple of pounds, check your portion sizes.

How serious this danger is can be illustrated by the fact that many insist it is the single biggest cause of the drive into obesity plaguing both our children and our society. Lisa Young, an author and researcher with New York University discussed this idea in a *USA Today* article,

> Studies show that the more food put in front of people, the more they eat. And since the 1960s, the serving sizes of foods sold in stores and restaurants—from candy bars to burgers and sodas—have become much bigger. . . .
>
> Others agree with Young's premise. "Portion distortion is a major contributor to many expanding waistlines," the American Heart Association reports."

Young then gives some examples of this portion creep: "Bagels used to be 2 to 3 ounces, or about 200 calories. Today they're 5 to 6 ounces, which is more than 400 calories." She concludes, "Don't buy into the idea that what the restaurant is serving you is an appropriate amount to eat. It's possible you're getting three to four servings of meat at one meal." As mentioned in this article, the American Heart Association's *No-Fad Diet* book suggests cutting portions by twenty-five percent.[8]

Most of the problems just covered are pretty well handled by following the basic rules of the RMR diet. If you can't measure it and determine how many calories it is within a fair degree of accuracy, don't eat it; don't go over your RMR limit; don't eat much less than your RMR limit.

Sure, at times, there has been something I wanted and wasn't able to figure out relatively closely how many calories it was. In those cases I estimate the calorie count at a little more than I think it really is. But I can't do this often or it happens daily and becomes a habit

Perhaps some of the best tips are offered in a *Reader's Digest* article.

> Consider the four-quarters rule. Mentally split your dinner plate into four quarters. The perfect meal has a starch dish in one quarter, a protein in the second quarter, and vegetables in the remaining two quarters. . . .

Use a smaller dish. This tip might sound ridiculous, but it works. First and most obvious is that you can't put as much food on, say, a salad plate. . . .

Keep the seconds far away. If you put the extra chicken or mashed potatoes on the table, all you have to do is reach over to get them. If they are back in the kitchen (and even better, already put away) you'll be less inclined to gobble food mindlessly.[9]

NOTES

1. Robert Nicolosi, PhD; Diane Becker, ScD, MPH; Patricia Elmer, PhD, RD; John Foreyt, PhD; Wahida Karmally, MS, RD; Katherine McManus, MS, RD; Lynne W. Scott, MA, RD; Marilyn F. Zukel, MS, RD; "American Heart Association Guidelines for Weight Management Programs for Healthy Adults," American Heart Association Subcommittee for Nutrition, 1994, http://www.americanheart.org/presenter/jhtml?identifier=1226.
2. Nutracheck weight loss, "Diet Plateau," *Nutracheck*, http://www.nutracheck.co.uk/Library/WeightLoss/diet-plateau_1.html.
3. "Plateau Buster Diet," ObesityHelp.com, http://www.obesityhelp.com/forums.
4. Pilkington, Nicky, "Diet Doldrums—Is Dehydration the Culprit?" Health-guidance.org, 2008, http://www.healthguidance.org/entry/5194/0/Diet-Doldrums---Is-Dehydration-the-Culprit.html.
5. Kennedy, Renee, "How to Break Out of a Weight Loss Plateau," About.com, http://thyroid.about.com/cs/dietweightloss/a/blplateau.htm?r=94.
6. Mayo Clinic, "Snacks: How they fit into your weight-loss plan," Mayo Foundation for Medical Education and Research, May 30, 2008, http://www.mayoclinic.com/health/healthy-diet/HQ01396.
7. AlinaBradford, "How To Make Your Own Diet Snack Packs," eHow, http://www.ehow.com/how_2136016_own-diet-snack-packs.html?ref=fuel&utm_source=y.
8. Hellmich, Nanci, "Portion Distortion," *USA Today*, http://www.usatoday.com/news/health/2005-06-21-portion-usat_x.htm.
9. Adapted from *The Everyday Arthritis Solution* by Richard Laliberte, "Practicing Proper Portions," Reader's Digest, http://www.rd.com/health/pain/nutrition-and-recipes-for-pain/practicing-proper-portions/article19011.html.

4

Nutrition

Socrates said, "Be aware the one and only secret to being healthy which has stood the test of time for optimum health and well being is healthy eating." The older we get the more we will realize that health is one of the most important things in life. That's what the RMR diet is all about.

It helps correct problems with obesity we have never thought about. For example, many of us think we can see our fat. But what we can see is only a part of the problem. Once we begin packing on the fat, our bodies start fattening up inside as well as out. Not only is this fat dangerous, but it is so insidious that even skinny people can have this kind of fat and not know it. One article explains this, "If it really is on the inside that counts, then a lot of thin people might be in trouble. Some doctors now think that the internal fat surrounding vital organs like the heart, liver, or pancreas—invisible to the naked eye—could be as dangerous as the more obvious external fat that bulges underneath the skin."[1]

We are used to thinking of our bodies as things that pretty well take care of themselves. Too often we forget that what we call a body is actually a wonderfully fine-tuned machine. The foods we eat and liquids we drink are nothing more than the means of fueling that machine with the chemicals and energy it needs to survive. What we call nutrition is, in the end, nothing more than thousands of chemical processes.

Our bodies are far more important to us than all of the other machines in our lives put together. All of us know that the machines in our lives need proper care, an adequate and dependable source of power or fuel, and occasional repair.

We change the filter bags on our vacuums, replace the tires on our cars, make sure our lawn mowers have gas and oil, and on, and on with every machine we own or use. We know we must do these things to keep those machines operating properly.

This analogy between a machine and a body can help us stay focused on the fact that certain mandatory care must be taken or a disastrous breakdown is inevitable. When such care is given, among the many other benefits is health.

Fuel for our bodies is measured in calories, just as fuel for our cars is measured in gallons. But there is a huge difference between the two sources of fuel. Besides fuel, the calories we eat must also contain all the vitamins, minerals, fiber, and protein that will keep our bodies from breaking down.

BALANCING YOUR NUTRITIONAL NEEDS

On a diet there are many things we must consider. For example, we cannot just focus on the amount of calories we eat. Sometimes we must consume higher calorie foods to maintain a nutritional balance. Protein, for example, is usually higher in calories than some other foods, but it is an essential nutrient. While we normally think of calcium as a prime necessity for building bones, protein plays a role in that process as well.

> Prevention of osteoporosis is a public health priority. Among nutritional factors, most attention has focused on the beneficial role of calcium and calcium-rich foods. . . . However, in addition to calcium, many other nutrients are necessary for bone health. Protein is critical for the skeleton. . . . Findings from many, but not all, epidemiological studies point to the beneficial role for dietary protein in bone health. . . . Low dietary protein intake has been associated with low bone mineral density and greater fracture risk in older adults.[2]

When it comes to building huge muscles, body builders are almost fanatic about increasing their protein intake. Not only is steak a favorite, but now protein-rich drinks flood the market, and their stomachs.

While the importance of protein to all parts of our lean body mass has been discussed, that is only a part of why we should be eating sufficient quantities of it. When we said hair and nails were not part of lean body mass, what we did not add was that they, too, are made of protein. "You need protein [to] build and maintain the structures of your body. Protein is also important for a healthy immune system, and for hormone production."[3]

Given all this, is it any wonder there are high-protein, low-carb diets that have been famous for decades? Many diets such as the Atkins, South Beach, Zone, Protein Buster, Sugar Buster, and Stillman diets insist that a diet high in protein and low on carbs is the way to go.

The American Heart Association asserts that "These [low-carb] diets can cause a quick drop in weight because eliminating carbohydrates causes a loss of body fluids. Lowering carbohydrate intake also prevents the body from completely burning fat. . . . But these diets have other effects besides inducing quick weight loss. . . . And eating too much protein can increase health risks."[4]

While this book is not about which other diets are good or bad, a recent study of the health problems some people reported might be worth consideration. The report is titled *Analysis of Health Problems Associated with High-Protein, High-Fat, Carbohydrate-Restricted Diets Reported via an Online Registry*. It was produced by the Physicians Committee for Responsible Medicine. Among other things, it says, "Mixed diets high in animal protein have been shown to increase the risk of kidney problems, osteoporosis, and some types of cancer."[5]

Part of the study was a well advertised website where people who had been on a high-protein, low-carb diet could register information about themselves and then log in health problems they have had. Here were the findings:

44 percent reported constipation

40 percent reported loss of energy

40 percent reported bad breath

29 percent reported difficulty concentrating

19 percent reported kidney problems: kidney stones (10 percent), severe kidney infections (1 percent), or reduced kidney function (8 percent)

33 percent reported heart-related problems, including 13 individuals reporting heart attack, stent placement, or bypass surgery, 26 reporting arrthymias, 42 reporting other cardiac problems, and 58 reporting elevated serum cholesterol levels

9 percent reported gallbladder problems or removal

5 percent reported gout
4 percent reported diabetes
4 percent reported colorectal (1 percent) or other cancers (3 percent)
3 percent reported osteoporosis[6]

And the news isn't much better on the high-carb, low-protein diet side of the fence. In a study of 1,866 women, "researchers interviewed the women about their diets and found that breast cancer risk rose with carbohydrate consumption." The article goes on to say that this one study is not definitive and more research needs to be done. "All carbohydrates are not alike. In this study, one kind particularly stood out—sucrose, or table sugar."[7]

It seems that for every study or opinion quoted, there are a dozen with opposing views. The majority of studies however, even ones for or against a particular side, point out that some carbs are good. The same was said about proteins.

The RMR diet favors neither protein nor carbs. Instead, by balancing your nutritional needs, the RMR diet promotes good health as well as weight loss.

In addition to protein and carbs, another food item that is extremely important in taking care of our bodies is fiber. Most of us know fiber is essential in preventing and treating constipation. What is not so well known is that it can help reduce hemorrhoids, diverticulosis, and is especially good in helping decrease cholesterol. "Different types of plants have varying amounts and kinds of fiber, including pectin, gum, mucilage, cellulose, hemicellulose and lignin."[8]

Another article gives some advice about including fiber in your diet and balancing your nutritional needs in general.

> Focus on fiber, . . . especially vegetables, fruit, beans, whole grains and fiber supplements. . . . Avoid fried foods. Bake, broil, or stir-fry (with very little oil) instead. Eat many mini-meals. Five or six small meals a day will help keep you from getting too hungry, control your blood sugar, and help you to eat fewer calories. . . . Drink lots of water. Pure water is healthy and filling with no added calories. Keep a journal. Use your food journal and calorie chart to keep track of calories. Some people also use a journal to better understand and manage emotions. Exercise daily. . . . Exercise improves metabolism.[9]

Gee, I couldn't have said it better myself. Jokes aside, all these things are at the heart of the RMR diet, and at the heart of what makes the diet so easy to do and to do so successfully.

SUPPLEMENTS

Whether dieting or not, food supplements such as vitamin and mineral tablets can go a long way in helping protect our health. In fact the holistic medicine field utilizes such items in many of their efforts to improve health. Every vitamin and mineral the body needs can be obtained by eating the right amounts, and the right types of food. But learning about what you need is complicated, confusing, and sometimes stressful since the health costs could be so drastic if certain nutrients are missing from your diet.

Almost all standard medical associations—such as the American Heart Association—assert that the best way to get proper nutrients is to have a proper diet. They then go on to quote some of the benefits dietary supplements can bring, but hedge their statements so as to not come right out and endorse them.

As with everything else in the RMR eating plan, what you do is up to you. If you have any doubts about whether you are getting proper nutrition, or if you have a problem that might be helped by taking supplements, you can research them on the internet yourself, or visit any reputable health food store for information specific to your circumstances. And, as with everything else, getting proper nutrition is up to you—however you do it.

As previously stressed, I am neither a doctor nor a dietician, but I do know that "moderation in all things" can be a guide here as well. When considering multivitamins, it seems those from natural sources are far better than the cheaper synthetic varieties. In fact, there are a number of studies that claim certain synthetic vitamins (such as ascorbic acid—vitamin C) may be harmful to one's health.

On 28th February 2007, the UK press reported on a study into synthetic vitamin and mineral supplements conducted at Copenhagen University.

The study found that money spent on such synthetic supplements was wasted and worse, they may increase mortality rates by 5 percent. The Diagnostic Clinic has always believed that synthetic (isolate structure) supplements could be dangerous in high doses and conferred little nutritional benefit, always recommending instead Food-State structure products which are as close to the natural food format as you can get.[10]

Since I am not a chemical researcher, either, I cannot elaborate on the scope or accuracy of that study. Being a writer, I look for words. "Can actually increase" does not mean "will increase." "Could be dangerous" does not mean "is always dangerous." I would, however not argue in any way with the fact that high doses of anything are not a good idea, including some of the medicines our doctors give us if we exceed the amount on the label.

MANAGING YOUR EMOTIONS

Emotional eating contributes greatly to the skyrocketing rates of obesity. It is another of those diet busters we have previously discussed.

One problem in controlling emotional eating, or even studying it is that there are so many types of emotional eating. A second problem is that under all the rest, your emotions are both a big part, and a measure, of who you are. Let's face it, emotional eating is such a part of us, we will all, at times, let our emotions cause us to overeat.

At best, all this book, any other book, a counselor, or a friend can do is offer suggestions about how to solve such emotional eating. Only you can discover where your own emotional dangers when it comes to food, and not let them cause you more difficulty. When it comes to dieting, the point is to control your emotions, not get rid of them. This can only be done by becoming aware of what your emotional eating problems are. Obviously, you can't possibly control something if you don't even know you're doing it. The Mayo Clinic published an invaluable resource for dealing with this problem.

> Sometimes the strongest longings for food happen when you're at your weakest point emotionally. Many people turn to food for comfort—consciously or unconsciously—when they're facing a difficult problem or looking to keep themselves occupied.
>
> But emotional eating—eating as a way to suppress or soothe negative emotions, such as stress, anger, anxiety, boredom, sadness and loneliness—can sabotage your weight-loss efforts. . . .
>
> The good news is that if you're prone to emotional eating, you can take steps to regain control of your eating habits and get back on

track. . . . Major life events such as unemployment, health problems and divorce—and daily life hassles—such as a stressful work commute, bad weather and changes to your normal routine—can trigger emotions that lead to overeating. But why do negative emotions lead to overeating?

Some foods may have seemingly addictive qualities. For example when you eat enticing foods, such as chocolate, your body releases trace amounts of mood and satisfaction elevating hormones. . . . Food can also be a distraction. If you're worried about an upcoming event or rethinking an earlier conflict, eating comfort foods may distract you . . .

Though strong emotions can trigger cravings for food, you can take steps to control those cravings. To help stop emotional eating, try these suggestions: Learn to recognize true hunger. Is your hunger physical or emotional? . . . If you . . . don't have a rumbling stomach, you're probably not really hungry. Give the craving a few minutes to pass.

Know your triggers. For the next several days, write down . . . how you're feeling when you eat and how hungry you are. Over time, you may see patterns emerge that reveal negative eating patterns and triggers to avoid.

Look elsewhere for comfort. Instead of unwrapping a candy bar, take a walk, treat yourself to a movie, listen to music, read or call a friend. If you think that stress relating to a particular event is nudging you towards the refrigerator, try talking to someone about it to distract yourself. Plan enjoyable events for yourself.

Don't keep unhealthy food around. . . . Snack healthy. . . . Eat a balanced diet. . . . Exercise regularly and get adequate rest.[11]

A HEALTHY WEIGHT

One final thing to consider regarding nutrition and health is the very weighty problem (pun intended) of when to shift from consuming your RMR to your BMR calories because you have lost all the weight you need to. Some things are obvious. Being too thin is unhealthy. Being obese is unhealthy. But where, in between, should you work to become?

Previously we covered Body Mass Index as a way of determining whether you are underweight, average weight, overweight, or obese. But BMI only gives an indication of whether you are at a weight that is healthy for you. Unfortunately, finding the exact right weight for a given individual is difficult for a variety of reasons. For example, "big athletes with lots of muscle might have a BMI over 30.0 but would not be considered obese from the perspective of health risk."[12] Furthermore, "people come in all different shapes and sizes, and the best weight for you is one that is right for your individual body type and size. It can be unhealthy to be too thin if you are eating less food than your body needs."[13]

Even the high fashion world is reconsidering the ideal body type. A *New York Times* journalist reported from Paris, "In the capital of high fashion and ultra thin models, conservative French legislators adopted a pioneering law Tuesday aimed at stifling a proliferation of Web sites that promote eating disorders with 'thinspiration' and starvation tips."[14]

And those are only some of the problems involved in deciding just where to shift your eating pattern from RMR to BMR. Another problem is that when most people picture the correct weight for themselves they frequently imagine how they want to look. This can be a useful tool as long as that picture is not the body type of an anorexic model on a fashion runway, or anything approaching it. Another useful tool is recognizing that being slightly overweight is not necessarily unhealthy. Far more important is if your weight is low enough to prevent the problems associated with being obese and if you are getting proper nutrition. Since your basal metabolism shrinks as you lose weight, if you are not careful you can get down to where maintaining proper nutrition is difficult.

In summation, here are two suggestions. The first is that you need not worry about this when beginning a diet. The second is that once the diet has eliminated a lot of your excess fat, it might be wise to consult with your doctor about what weight would be healthiest for you.

THE DANGERS OF POOR NUTRITION

It cannot be stressed enough that losing too much weight can be very unhealthy if nutrition suffers. In the end, obesity is simply poor nutrition by consuming too many calories. We have also covered the importance of adhering as closely as you can to the food pyramid for your own particular stage in life.

When someone brings up the financial cost of being overweight, for example, we tend to think about how much the extra food is costing us. That is considerable, yet we rarely even give a thought to how being overweight or obese is affecting both our own finances, and the finances of the nation.

One article says, "The latest studies estimate that obesity alone costs the US around $75 billion annually." In addition it asserts, "On an individual level, obesity increases annual medical spending per person by 37.4 percent, or around $730 a year. And overweight increases spending per person by 14.5 percent, or $247 per year."[15] Perhaps, for a millionaire, these costs are not significant. But to most of us having to pay the piper for all that extra food we put in our mouth is only a small part of the costs.

In addition to all the other ways losing weight will help us, taking care of our bodies can bring tremendous financial benefits. While going on the RMR diet will not make you rich, it certainly can cut down your cost of living.

However, there will probably be a slight cost increase due to some of your changes in diet. The great value of eating more fruits and vegetables in terms of vitamins, minerals, and satisfying hunger has already been covered. However, the costs of these foods in relation to the higher carb and protein foods is rising. "Recent studies show that the cost of high-calorie foods are less likely to be affected by inflation and, on average, cost less than low-calorie foods."[16] On the other hand, a pound of broccoli hardly compares with the cost of a pound of sirloin. Whatever the cost, in the long run, taking care of your health is far cheaper than neglecting it.

For the average person, far more important than the monetary costs of healthy foods are the health costs of not spending what we must to maintain our health. For instance, there is the matter of maintaining your longevity. How long do you want your machine to last? How can you make it last longer? How can you get more health, activity, and happiness during those added years? Finding good answers to these questions is what the RMR diet is all about.

NOTES

1. Maria Cheng, "Diet: Thin people may be fat inside," Associated Press, as published online in the Boston Globe, May 10, 2007, http://www.boston.com/yourlife/health/diseases/articles/2007/05/10/diet_thin_people_may_be_fat_inside/ (accessed Aug 27, 2008).

2. Dairy Council, "Dietary protein & Bone Health: New perspectives," Dairy Council Digest Archives, http://www.nationaldairycouncil.org/NationalDairyCouncil/Health/Digest/dcd74-5Page1.html.

3. Jegtvig, Shereen, "Improve Your Nutrition One Day at a Time," About.com, March 2, 2009, http://nutrition.about.com/od/nutritiontips/qt/dnt222.htm.

4. American Heart Association, "High-Protein Diets," American Heart Association, Inc., http://www.americanheart.org/presenter.jhtml?identifier=11234.

5. Neal D. Barnard, M.D. and Amy Jo Lanou, Ph.D, "Analysis of Health Problems Associated with High-Protein, High-Fat, Carbohydrate-Restricted Diets Reported via an Online Registry" Physicians Committee for Responsible Medicine, May 25, 2004, http://www.pcrm.org/health/reports/highprotein_registry.html.

6. Ibid.

7. Miranda Hitti, reviewed by Brunilda Nazario, MD, "High-Carb Diet Linked to Breast Cancer," WebMD Medical News, August 6, 2004, http://www.webmd.com/content/article/92/101647.htm.

8. J. Anderson, S. Perryman, L. Young, and S. Prior, "*Dietary Fiber*," Colorado State University Extension, http://www.ext.colostate.edu/pubs/foodnut/09333.html.

9. Moss Greene, "Food Calorie Chart of Healthy Foods," BellaOnline, http://www.bellaonline.com/articles/art44090.asp.

10. Rajendra Sharma, "TDC Press release on the dangers of synthetic vitamins and mineral supplements," The Diagnostic Clinic, http://www.thediagnosticclinic.com/dangers percent20of percent20synthetic percent20vitamin percent20and percent20mineral percent20supplements.htm.

11. Mayo Clinic Staff, "Weight-loss help: How to stop emotional eating," Mayo Foundation for Medical Research, http://www.mayoclinic.com/health/weight-loss/MH00025.

12. "Learn About Body Mass Index (BMI)," National Heart Lung and Blood Institute, http://www.nhlbi.nih.gov/health/public/heart/obesity/wecan/learn-it/bmi-chart.htm.

13. Mary L. Gavin, MD, "What's the Right Weight for Me?" KidsHealth, The Nemours Foundation, May 2005, http://kidshealth.org/kid/talk/qa/fat_thin.html.

14. Doreen Carvajal, "French bill takes aim at extreme thinness," *Salt Lake Tribune*, April 16, 2008.

15. Jessica Branom-Zwick, "Medical Cost of Obesity," *Sightline Daily*, August 17, 2005, http://daily.sightline.org/daily_score/archive/2005/08/17/medical_cost_of/?searchterm=overweight.

16. Stacy Kish, "Healthy, Low-Calorie Foods Cost More on Average," United States Department of Agriculture: Cooperative State Research, Education, and Extension Service, March 19, 2008, http://www.csrees.usda.gov/newsroom/impact/2008/nri/03191_food_prices.html.

5

Ways to Burn Calories

There are 3600 calories in a pound of fat. That's the way we usually look at it. More accurately, a pound of fat releases 3600 calories of heat when the body uses it. A pound of oil contains 3600 calories, the same as a pound of fat. On a daily diet of two thousand calories you will burn the equivalent of fifty five percent of that pound of oil per day.

That's what metabolism is all about, a measurement of the amount of heat your body uses each day. The higher your metabolism, the more heat you use. And the more heat you use, the more fat you have to burn to supply that heat.

Before we start looking at ways to raise metabolism and get the benefits of doing so in some depth, the article *How Do I Raise My Metabolism*, gives a quick overview; here are some of the more common ways to raise your metabolism it mentions.

> Weight training itself has been shown to increase exercise post oxygen consumption (EPOC)—in other words, your metabolism may be raised for hours, or even days, after the session. . . .
>
> Do you play the game of driving around the parking lot for twenty minutes waiting for the perfect space to open? Instead, park at the edge of the parking lot and walk to your destination. You'll probably get there quicker, and burn some calories along the way. Other metabolism-boosting activities include standing instead of sitting, taking stairs instead of elevators, and even fidgeting![1]

The article then goes on to list some additional ideas for raising your metabolism. It says, "don't fear carbohydrates," "increase protein," "perform high-intensity cardio," "increase frequency of eating," "eat whole foods," and "drink cold water." These suggestions generally increase your metabolism by increasing the calories you use. Even relatively short bursts of activity will boost your metabolism for the next twenty-four hours.[2]

We cannot overlook the added value more activity brings in boosting our health.

> Regular exercise and physical activity are extremely important and beneficial for long-term health and well-being. . . .
>
> [The] health benefits of exercise and physical activity [include the following]: reduce the risk of premature death; reduce the risk of developing and/or dying from heart disease; reduce high blood pressure or the risk of developing high blood pressure; reduce high cholesterol or the risk of developing high cholesterol; reduce the risk of developing colon cancer and breast cancer; reduce the risk of developing diabetes; reduce or maintain body weight or body fat; build and maintain healthy muscles, bones, and joints; reduce depression and anxiety; improve psychological well-being; enhance work, recreation and sport performance.[3]

But since this book is also about losing weight, a short look at how different activities burn calories is also useful. Remember, while the study that will be quoted is for a one hundred fifty pound person doing the various activities for a half hour, if you weigh more, you will be burning more calories for each activity.

Also, since a pound of fat is 3600 calories, if you want to know how many hours you would have to do a certain activity to burn a pound, double the amount shown and divide it into 3600. Another thing you might want to calculate is just how many days of doing that activity it takes to burn the pound of fat. This is especially important because any activity engaged in numerous times per week over a long period of time is far more effective than short bursts of that activity. Note the following list of calories burned by an average 150-pound person for each half hour of a given activity.[4]

Activity	Calories burned
Walking (3.5 mph; 17 min/mile)	170
Jogging (6 mph; 10 min/mile)	450
Cycling (12–14 mph; moderate effort)	360
Swimming (laps, vigorously)	450
Aerobics (moderate effort)	275
Yard Work or House Work	225
Strength Training (moderate)	200
Stretching	115
Yoga (moderate)	150
Office Work (Sitting)	70
Office Work (Standing)	100
Sleeping	40

One of the things these figures bring up is that strength training uses fewer calories than house or yard work. This is not intended to disparage going to the gym, using weights at home, or doing other sorts of strength training. Without doubt, on a weight loss program such exercises build muscle mass, and we've already covered how that increases metabolism.

It is intended, however, to show that many things we don't normally consider exercise (like house and yard work) are in fact exercise and help the fat disappear. And whether it be one of the more vigorous forms of exercise, or a regular exercise such as walking three or more times per week, exercise is certainly recommended highly. Obviously, the best results will be gained by exercising nearly every day for at least half an hour. But even just three days a week can help to maintain your hearts and lungs.

STRETCHING

Another fairly easy type of exercise that has great benefits is bending and stretching. Look at your dog or cat if you have one, you will see that stretching even helps your pet. Stretching is almost instinctual. Ever stretch when you yawn? How about when you get out of bed in the morning?

Stretching is one of those things that, if done properly, can and should be performed by any age group. It is extremely important when engaging in any sport or another form of exercise, including walking. And it is one of the most highly recommended activities for seniors.

"Stretching is a form of physical exercise in which a specific skeletal muscle (or muscle group) is deliberately elongated to its fullest length . . . in order to improve the muscle's felt elasticity and reaffirm comfortable muscle tone. The result is a feeling of increased muscle control, flexibility and range of motion."[5]

In short, stretching improves muscle tone and increases flexibility. And, like everything else, if you're well motivated, you could begin a daily stretching program. But, as with anything you do on the RMR diet, even a small amount of stretching brings good results—and burns calories.

No matter how much or how little stretching you do, there are a few things you should remember.

> Stretching exercises are thought to give you more freedom of movement to do the things you need to do and the things you like to do. Stretching exercises alone will not improve your endurance or strength . . .

> If you can't do endurance or strength exercises for some reason, and stretching exercises are the only kind you are able to do, do them at least 3 times a week, for at least 20 minutes each session. . . . Do stretching exercise 3 to 5 times at each session.

> Slowly stretch into the desired position as far as possible without pain, and hold the stretch for 10 to 30 seconds. Relax, then repeat, trying to stretch farther. . . . Stretching should never cause pain, especially joint pain. If it does, you are stretching too far, and you need to reduce the stretch so that it doesn't hurt. Mild discomfort or a mild pulling sensation is normal. Never "bounce" into a stretch; make slow, steady movements instead. Jerking into position can cause muscles to tighten, possibly resulting in injury.

> Avoid "locking" your joints into place when you straighten them during stretches. Your arms and legs should be straight when you stretch them, but don't lock them in a tightly straight position. You should always have a very small amount of bending in your joints while stretching.[6]

If stretching is something you really want to get into, there are a number of helpful books, web sites, and videos to guide you.[7]

Unconcious Fat Burning

If you are one of those who do weight training, vigorous exercise, or regular aerobic exercise, good for you—keep it up. You probably already know the importance of stretching as part of your exercise routine to help prevent injury. If you are seriously planning to engage in weight training or vigorous exercise, good for you—get to it. But if your health or time of life makes doing such things difficult right now, read on.

Think about it for a moment. Standing up burns fat. Sitting back down burns fat. Eating burns fat. Putting your hands behind your head burns fat. Every single thing you do burns fat if your caloric intake does not exceed your RMR limit.

Allow me to share my own experiences with activity. They may provide some useful information, no matter what stage of life or activity level you are currently experiencing. Many tasks I do at my age are no longer pleasurable. I used to enjoy being out in the sun cutting my lawn. Shoveling snow was equally enjoyable when I was dressed warmly, at least at the start of winter. But now the only satisfaction I find in doing such things is that I can still do them.

When I first started the RMR diet, every time I climbed the stairs in my house, the fact that I was burning calories came to mind. Ditto while I was helping my wife, Bobbie, by vacuuming. The same for walking the dogs or just swinging on our porch swing.

Everything I did now had an extra dimension. I actually began to find joy again in doing what had long since become routine tasks. Every single one of them was helping my calorie-burning efforts. This was such a thrill, I could not forget that what I was doing meant burning those calories. Most amazing was that I began looking for tasks to do that would help the weight drop.

Soon, however, this degree of motivation was replaced by an even greater one that occurred when I finally realized that what I was burning was not calories. I was burning fat. What a realization! The calories I thought I was burning were just the measurement of how much I'd have to do to get rid of one more pound.

Physiologists tell us that the structure of the human body was created by standing and walking. Therefore, sitting is one of the unhealthy things we do to ourselves. For example, any occupation that requires a person to sit for long periods of time, like working at a computer all day, has health risks. Is it any wonder many of us have back problems, not to mention all the other problems that long periods of sitting create?

One of these risks is the metabolic syndrome. An online article geared toward women asks, "Sitting at a desk or in front of a computer for hours a day, spending hours in the car running the kids around, grabbing dinner on the run and collapsing at the end of the day. Sound like your life? If so, you could be one of the millions of women who are at risk for developing the metabolic syndrome, a cluster of risk factors for heart disease and diabetes. A 'syndrome' means that this is a collection of health risks, not a disease itself." [9]

After reading this article, I knew I was risking the metabolic syndrome by sitting and watching TV. A commercial came on and I began thinking of some other activity I could do to burn more fat. Then, I discovered a plan that went beyond anything I had previously considered to burn that fat.

We are told that inactivity is one of the worst enemies of any weight loss program. Yet that is exactly what I was doing. I was totally inactive during a TV program. I spent the commercials only thinking of how I could burn fat. Then I got it! I could change doing nothing into doing something by simply getting up during the commercials and doing anything!

How simple. In a few hours of watching TV, I'm watching dozens of commercials in three to five minute time periods. Doing something during that time, for, say, two or three programs each day could boost my fat burning ability greatly. And it really doesn't matter how little the something I do is. If I just get up and sit back down during those commercials, I have not only burned a lot of calories, I've strengthened my leg muscles.

If this doesn't seem like much, consider this. There are approximately eighteen commercial breaks during two hours of programming. That's 126 times per week we can get up. In a year that comes to 6552 times more you will get up instead of just sitting there. Still think getting up during commercials is nothing?

Since you are raising the number of pounds you weigh every time you get up, if you weigh 150 pounds you will have raised 490 tons of body weight in that first year. If you weigh 200 pounds you will raise 655 tons! Don't believe me? Do the math yourself.

Doing this during commercial breaks is great, but it's not the only way. If, for example, you don't watch TV a lot, but read every day, get up and do something every half hour or at the end of every chapter. Is playing video games your thing? Pick a set number of games you play and then get up and do something.

Remember, the greatest muscle mass on our bodies lies below our waist lines. Since those are our largest muscle masses, it makes a lot of sense that our quickest and easiest way to build our basic metabolic rate is to strengthen and build those muscles. The increase of metabolism from building these muscles is so substantial that, in fact, it can even surpass the increased metabolism accomplished in strength training to increase our arm size.

Now count the steps you might take if you moved around after you got up. Then add in any other activity you might engage in, and it is no wonder that we can truly achieve considerable health building and fat burning from avoiding something that most of us don't like any way.

Among the many ways I've suggested you might get better results from this RMR diet, I am now recommending that if you are not already engaging in sufficient exercise routines, try the "no commercial" form of exercise.

Why is doing something when TV commercials come on advocated instead of just promoting something like standing up more during the day? I don't know about your mental functions, but I find I often need reminders to do something I know I should be doing. From now on every time you see a commercial, you can be reminded you can improve your life by no longer just sitting there on your recliner.

A further reason commercial non-watching was chosen is that we do not want our new way of life to replace things beneficial, enjoyable, or otherwise worthwhile in our lives. Few amongst us would claim watching commercials is a powerful force for enjoyment. Fewer still would argue that watching fewer commercials would in anyway impoverish us. Thus, getting some commercials out of our lives is a bonus in and of itself.

Yet another reason commercial non-watching was chosen: advertisers will hate this whole concept. If you watch fewer commercials, you may end up not buying something you didn't want or need in the first place.

There is that old adage, "Use it or lose it." Not only will we not be losing it, the No Commercial exercise plan will make us better at using "it" because a habit practiced is a habit reinforced. Since this habit results in increased energy, we have more energy and ability to engage in those other things in life that we enjoy! If nothing else came of it, this would still make this program something fruitful.

But there is also a loss. Let's take a look at what we'll be losing. We'll be losing the many benefits advertisers promise if we'll only buy everything that is being pawned off on us in those commercials. What a loss! Possibly we will also be losing all the useful information and knowledge commercials provide us with ten or twelve times during a short program. Sorry, sometimes I can't help being sarcastic when it comes to commercials. Well, maybe I can help it. But being cantankerous about certain things can be fun at my age.

One caution when you first begin doing this: you must let significant others know what you're doing when you really get serious at this. When my sister Glenda started on the program, she didn't tell her husband what she was going to do. About the third time she got up and did something during a commercial, her husband, Larry, asked, "What, in heaven's name, are you doing now?"

Also, don't put commercials on mute when you get up because you will miss your program when the commercial ends. In fact you might want to turn the volume up louder when you're going into another room if you can do so without disturbing someone else.

One thing I know about myself is that I have a long history of starting vast projects with half vast ideas. How else could a person lose over a thousand pounds as I have on the many diet programs I have tried? The problem has always been eventually getting worn down by it all and reverting to my self-destructive eating habits and periods of decreased activity.

So, I vowed that for the first three weeks I would limit myself to letting the commercials remind me to get up and do something to a single half-hour program. It didn't matter what I did as long as I got up and did it. And I could even do something I enjoyed doing! It was so exhilarating I immediately jumped to an hour program and did that for three weeks to start. So, it actually took me over a month to get to the two hour a day goal.

I must report, however, that as my energy level grew, I sometimes began doing things I enjoyed much more than to finish watching the current program I had been viewing. Not watching so much TV? Horrors. That's almost as bad as the very real possibility that if we don't see something the advertisers are peddling, we won't be tempted to buy it.

Another tip: before you start each day, use your senses and look around. You might want to make a short list of things you could do during commercials. Put down regular tasks you have postponed or that need doing now. If something looks bad or looks out of place, put it on the list. Keep it fairly short, and keep the tasks you list simple.

Finally, do not discount what can be accomplished during these short commercial breaks. Years ago, when four hundred dollars was a lot of money, I spent that much for a "More Time" workshop. I got a few lessons from the program that have helped make my life more productive. The presenter's first words were, "There is no such thing as more time. Everyone is allowed only sixty seconds to a minute. Everything you can possibly do can only be accomplished minute by minute. You can all go home now. I've given you your money's worth if you will learn the truth of this." During the course of the workshop, I also learned that the greatest waster of that time is not finishing what I start.

In case you don't consider just taking more steps during the day as an exceptionally valuable way to burn fat and improve our health, consider the following from Laurie Barclay, MD: "Instructing sedentary women to walk 10,000 steps per day is more effective at increasing exercise per day than is asking them to walk 30 minutes on most days of the week, according to a randomized study published in the April [2005] issue of *Medicine and Science in Sports and Exercise*." She went on to say this same result can be achieved by men.[8]

Previously I recommended obtaining a pedometer. Now this advice can be better understood. The whole point is that the number of steps you take during a day is what matters, not whether you take them all at once as in a walk, or just in your activities during the day. Naturally, a brisk walk will also have cardio-vascular benefits.

By hooking a pedometer to your waist in the morning for a couple of days, and then reading and recording it at night, you can discover how many steps your normal day uses. Then all you need do is increase it to the suggested number.

One of the most common reasons we don't do something is that some tasks just seem overwhelming. We believe it will take too much time and too much energy to get it done. A good way to overcome these seemingly overwhelming tasks is to tell ourselves we will work on it, but not for more than a few minutes at a time—about the length of a commercial break. Once we have spent a few of these short periods "punching holes" in any task that has been nagging at us, it will no longer be so overwhelming and finishing it will be much simpler. The workshop called this extremely useful process, "Swiss cheezing it."

Here are just a few tasks that might be Swiss cheezed either because they are overwhelming or simply can't be accomplished during one commercial break. Begin sweeping a room; quit when your program comes on, then begin again at the next set of commercials. Begin vacuuming the room; shut off the vacuum when your program comes on, then begin again at the next set of commercials. Begin straightening up a closet, cupboard, or drawer.

Even Simpler Activities:

Get up and pace around a little bit.
Just stand up during part of each commercial session.
Climb a set of stairs a couple of times.

Many people are motivated emotionally when working with others. At one point I joined a weight loss class at the YWCA. It worked—as long as I was going—and that's not bad.

The problem for me was that when I no longer had that "support group," the benefits I had achieved faded fast. This was because, whether I realized it or not, I was drawing power from them and not depending on my own power. Further, part of my motivation was to show others I could do it, or at least not let them see me fail.

All that being said, if you enjoy doing things with others, by all means share this program with them and get them enrolled in doing it with you. The same goes for a walking group, an aerobic group, or any other type of group that assists you.

Just remember, in the end, it is your power, and your power alone that will carry you on to this new and better life. The steps you take are up to you. As this next quote illustrates, you are the one in control.

> Americans have poured themselves into dieting for decades. From Atkins to South Beach to Fat Busters, we've actually spent the gross national product of Ireland each year on trying to slim down. It turns out it was free all along . . .
> What nobody talks about is that being healthy is not a matter of dieting, it is a matter of changing your life forever, eating healthy forever, moving your body, everyday, forever. No one wants to talk about that because it scares people to have that much control.[11]

NOTES

1. "How Do I Raise My Metabolism?" Natural Physiques, http://www.naturalphysiques.com/faq/458.html.

2. In discussing this, Wayne Mcgregor has posted an online article in which he asks, "Can you raise the metabolic rate without long exercise sessions? . . . The answer is yes!" To learn more about this phenomenon, read the full article: Wayne Mcgregor, "Raising the Metabolism with Little Exercise," EzineArticles.com, http://ezinearticle.com/?Raising-the-Metabolism-with-Little-Exercise&id=640193.

3. J. Andrew Doyle, PhD, *Health Benefits of Exercise*," Georgia State University, http://www2.gsu.edu/~wwwfit/benefits.html.

4. "Benefits of Exercise," *General Electric: My Health,* http://www.ge.com/myhealth/us/hbn_ten_exercise.html.

5. "Stretching," Wikipedia, http://en.wikipedia.org/wiki/Stretching.

6. "Chapter 4: Exercise Examples—Stretching Exercises," http://weboflife.nasa.gov/exerciseandaging/chapter4_stretching.html.

7. If you want to find some simple stretches to do, some of which you can even do sitting down, go to *Stretching and Flexibility Exercises* on www.americanheart.org.

8. "Metabolic Syndrome," http://my.clevelandclinic.org/heart/women/metabolic.aspx.

9. Laurie Barclay, "Step Counting May Increase Exercise More Than Timed Walking," http://cme.medscape.com/viewarticle/502693.

10. "Separating Fact from Fiction in the Age of Obesity," http://www.alternet.org/healthwellness/52196/?page=entire.

6

Calories and Portion Control

WATCHING YOUR PORTIONS

We have already discussed "portion creep," "super-sizing," and the problems associated with eating too much of any one type of food. Such things as getting smaller portions in restaurants and cutting down the portion sizes listed on nutritional labels have also been covered. Now comes an extremely important part of dieting—cooking. This is where we have the most control over calories and portions, because cooking is an ideal time to implement adherence to the food pyramid. In fact, the best time to do this is when you start taking your pots and pans out of the cupboard.

Even if you don't do the cooking in your home, knowing the information in this chapter can benefit you greatly. Or let's say you get a lot of your food while on the run. This information will still be useful to you. (Incidentally, it would probably behoove you to cut that wherever possible in favor of home cooking. For one thing, you can control your portions better at home.) If you don't do the cooking yourself, making occasional suggestions such as, "If it's all right, I think I'd like some broccoli for dinner," might be useful. Maybe bringing home some broccoli because "it was on sale," might work even better.

Many people who have to cook know that it can be both enjoyable and rewarding. When I am cooking something special I enjoy anticipating how it will taste, or planning to share it with others. Another time I enjoy cooking is when I do it with others, such as preparing a large holiday feast.

61

One of my specialties is a shrimp cocktail my mother taught me. Sadly, with our hectic lifestyles, these days it often seems that cooking is just another chore that needs to be done. It's a real shame that something so important can't be lingered over like in the old days.

First on the list of things to consider is portion control. If others in your family have weight problems, you might slowly cut down the amount you cook—very slowly. If you're the only one watching your RMR, cook normally for everyone else, but only include whatever amount you will be allowed to eat in addition to what you cook for everyone else.

One problem with portion control is not knowing the difference between a portion and a serving. "A 'portion' is how much food you choose to eat, whether in a restaurant, from a package, or in your own kitchen. A 'serving' is a standard amount set by the U.S. Government. . . . There are two commonly used standards for serving sizes: MyPyramid Plan . . . [and the] Food and Drug Administration (FDA) Nutrition Fact label."[1]

Understanding this difference helps keep in mind that the "serving size" on a package label does not tell you how much you should eat. It tells you how many calories and nutrients each serving contains. The pyramid tells you how many servings you should be getting.

THE JOYS (AND DANGERS) OF COOKING

How do we make sure we're getting the portions we should be getting when we're cooking? Back to the measuring spoons, cups, and scale. The scale is especially important when cooking. Many foods, hamburger for example, doesn't even have labels to guide us. To count the calories in these foods, use the scale to measure the ounces you've chosen as a portion, then look the calories up in a calorie book.

It will not be necessary to weigh, measure, and look up every bite you eat for the rest of your life. You need only do this long enough to recognize how big your portions are, what the approximate calorie count of them is, and how much you should be eating for proper nutrition.

There are plenty of websites that give helpful ways to estimate some things when you are no longer measuring exact amounts. For example, "1 medium fruit equals a baseball; ½ cup of fresh fruit equals ½ a baseball; 1 ½ ounces of low-fat or fat-free cheese equals 4 stacked dice; 2 tablespoons of peanut butter equals a ping-pong ball." [2]

Here are some more in-depth examples:

- 1 pancake—a compact disc (CD)
- 1 cup of pasta—a fist
- 1 cup potatoes, rice, pasta—a tennis ball
- 1 cup green salad—a baseball or a fist
- ½ cup serving—6 asparagus spears, 7 or 8 baby carrots or carrot sticks, or 1 ear of corn on the cob
- ¼ cup raisins—a large egg
- an ounce of cheese—a pair of dice or your thumb
- 1 cup of ice cream—a large scoop the size of a baseball
- 3 ounces cooked meat, fish, poultry—a palm, a deck of cards, or a cassette tape
- 2 tablespoons salad dressing—a ping-pong ball
- 1 teaspoon butter, margarine—size of a stamp, the thickness of your finger or a thumb tip
- 1 ½ cups of pasta, noodles—a dinner plate, not heaped[3]

Another thing to consider is how much to cook. We must often cook more than we'll use at one meal. It's hard to eat a large roast, turkey, or ham at one sitting unless you have several people to help you. You only have two choices: cook part of it or cook all of it. Cooking only part of something has a number of drawbacks: it takes more time to cook it later; using your stove twice is an inefficient use of energy; and let's not forget the time it takes to clean up after a second, or third, cooking of something that could easily be cooked only once.

There are also many things you might want (or need) to cook in larger amounts. When you do, you should already be familiar with the safety rules for storing excess food in a way that will keep it from spoiling. But instead of storing the leftovers in bulk, consider splitting them up into different containers (such as baggies or plastic bowls) in the portions you or the family will use to stay on your RMR plan.

Let's look at a few scenarios for how this might work in real life:

Scenario one: There's half a cup of sauce left over, what to do? It's such a small amount, I might as well eat it. (I've lost track of how often I've ruined a diet after a few such instances.)

Scenario two: "Hey, I've got about a quarter of a cup of sauce left. Anybody want more?" (This puts weight on others.)

Scenario three: I reach the pan over to the sink, close my eyes, and turn on the water, and start it into the pan. I open my eyes, and pour the partially filled pan into the garbage disposal.

After considering how much you need to prepare, and how many calories each thing contains, you're ready to head for the stove. So, what else will you have to think about? You will still want to consider your cooking methods and the additional ingredients each of them will require.

First, you had better use olive oil or peanut oil because they are more heart healthy. And probably it would work to use only one tablespoon instead of the four the recipe calls for. Let's see, how should you cook this? Most cooks already know that the way something is cooked can either increase or decrease its calories. For example, baking is lower in calories than frying, but baked eggs? One article explains how your cooking method can affect a certain dish's calories.

> Cooking low-calorie, low-fat dishes may not take a long time, but best intentions can be lost with the addition of butter or other added fats at the table. It is important to learn how certain ingredients can add unwanted calories and fat to low-fat dishes—making them no longer lower in calories and lower in fat!
>
> These cooking methods tend to be lower in fat: bake, broil, microwave, roast—for vegetables and/or chicken without skin, steam, lightly stir-fry or saute in cooking spray . . . grill seafood, chicken or vegetables. [4]

If popcorn is a favorite snack, use an air popper or non-buttered popcorn in your microwave. Then you can spray it with a non-fat butter spray. At the supermarket don't confuse "cholesterol-fat free" with fat free. Either kind contains the same amount of calories. Cholesterol free is just better for your arteries and your heart.

Another popular cooking method, especially in the summer months, is grilling. This next article gives detailed information about how to reduce your calories while grilling.

> Summer is a great time to break out the barbeque and lighten up your diet! Grilling season doesn't have to only mean hamburgers, bratwurst, and steaks. There are many great choices for the grill that will keep you in great shape for all those fun summer activities.
>
> Rather than fatty hunks of meat or sausages try grilling:
>
> —Chicken breast
>
> —Turkey breast or tenderloin

—Ground turkey, chicken, or lean hamburger (add great seasonings)

—Veggie/grain/or soy burgers

—Vegetables

—Turkey hot dogs or sausages/brats

—Fish (salmon, swordfish, shrimp, catfish, trout, red snapper, tuna, and so forth.)

—Or, if you choose beef, select a high-quality but small portion.

Marinades are easy to make and allow you to use some creativity in your cooking! If you're making your own marinade, plan on about a half cup per pound of meat. There are usually 3–4 components to a marinade. You'll definitely need an acid such as citrus juices, vinegars, or wine. This acid will serve to break down protein tissues in the meat, which will serve to tenderize. For flavor, you need to include some oil (canola, olive, sesame, or other) and seasonings (salt and pepper, dried or fresh herbs, soy sauce, Worcestershire sauce, ketchup, mustards, garlic, gingerroot, onion, chili peppers, etc.) You also might want to add a sugary ingredient like honey, jam, or molasses to add a touch of sweetness and carmelization to your grilled food. About a quarter to a third of the marinade should be the acid, a few tablespoons should be oil, about a tablespoon of your sugar ingredient, and seasonings can really be however much you like.

Make sure to always marinate in the refrigerator. Large zipper bags are great for marinating. Otherwise, use a shallow glass or plastic container. Avoid metal which will react with the acid in the marinade. . . . [Marinating] will also cut down a little bit on cooking times. Depending on what you're marinating, the times will vary. Here are some general rules to follow:

—Large cuts of meat (over 4 pounds)—8 hours to overnight

—Smaller cuts of meat—½ to 3 hours

—Whole fish—3 hours to overnight

—Fillets of fish (depending on size)—1 hour to overnight

—Fruits and vegetables—1 to 3 hours

Don't use leftover marinade for basting or as a sauce, unless you first boil it for 5 minutes to kill any bacteria. To prevent food from sticking to the grill, lightly coat your grilling surface with a small amount of cooking oil or spray. Some companies now make nonstick sprays specifically for the grill.[5]

When it comes to cooking higher fat items such as ham or a rump roast, the whole process can begin when you buy the meat. Inspecting different packages in the case will quickly evidence those that contain more fat, and those that have less fat on them. Then, before the meat is cooked even more fat can be trimmed off. A quick note: I find it easier to cut off the fat on a roast or a ham after I've cooked it.

When making gravy with the liquid from a pot roast, or a roast cooked in a Crock-Pot, the liquid should not be used right away. If it is poured off, put into a bottle and placed in the fridge, all the fat in it will congeal into a white cap on top of the liquid, which can then be easily removed. If you are in a hurry to use the liquid, putting it in the freezer will help it to congeal more quickly.

One final note about cooking is something that was mentioned earlier: there are many cooking lite cookbooks and the Internet is full of recipes. While many of the tips for cooking lite have already been covered, there are many, many more. If you're new to this type of cooking the sources mentioned in this chapter are almost a must.

SUGAR AND SWEETENERS

Without question, you can cut down on calories when cooking by the use of sugar substitutes, as this next article explains.

An easy way to cut back on calories without feeling deprived is to cook or bake with artificial sweeteners. You can shave 360 calories from a cake recipe that calls for 1 cup of sugar by using an artificial sweetener if place of half of it. (You can't replace *all* the sugar with a substitute. Start by replacing half, and if the food doesn't brown correctly, or is too heavy in texture, increase the sugar to sweetener ratio.) Not all substitutes will do for baking.

Sweet One: 4 calories per packet—12 packets = 1 cup sugar, 1 packet = 2 teaspoons sugar. Can be used in cooking and baking without losing sweetness.

Equal: 4 calories per packet—24 packets = 1 cup sugar; 1 packet = 2 teaspoons sugar. Loses sweetness when baked at high temperatures for a long time. Can be used in stir-fries or added during the last few minutes of heating or cooking. Equal has developed some baked recipes to use the sweetener with no breakdown. Visit website for recipes.

Equal Spoon Full: 2 calories per teaspoon—1 cup = 1 cup sugar; 1 teaspoon = 1 teaspoon sugar. Loses sweetness when heated to high temperatures for long periods of time. Can be used spoon for spoon in place of sugar in same foods as Equal. Equal has developed some baked recipes to use the sweetener with no breakdown. Visit website for recipes.

Splenda: 0 calories—1 cup = 1 cup sugar; 1 teaspoon = 1 teaspoon sugar. May not work well in recipes such as certain cakes that rely upon sugar for structure. Finished recipes may require refrigeration. See website for further details.

Sweet 'N Low: 4 calories per packet—12 packets = 1 cup sugar; 1 packet = 2 teaspoons sugar. Can be used in cooking and baking without loosing sweetness.

Brown Sweet 'N Low: 20 calories per teaspoon—4 teaspoons = 1 cup brown sugar. Can be used in cooking or baking without losing sweetness. Note that measurements differ from packet sweeteners.[6]

You can also reduce the sugar and carbohydrates in foods by substituting brown sugar or fruit juice. Honey supplies other nutrients along with its sweetness, which sometimes makes it a more appealing option. As was mentioned before, even Hershey has come up with a sugar-free chocolate.

Sugar, in and of itself, and in small amounts, is not necessarily bad. The problem is that it is included in so many foods for no useful purpose. This means you need to be vigilant about the number of foods you cook with sugar, especially because if sugar is used in a number of them, the communicative total of the sugar you are consuming may be quite high.

On the other hand, sweetness is such an important part of both our enjoyment of food and view of life, it is even synonymous with the good things in life. "Oh, isn't she sweet?" "She's my sweetheart." "Sweeter than life itself." So, you should not completely cut out those sweet things. Just make them more sugar free. This is just one more way to make the RMR eating process more comfortable.

As mentioned, the amount of oil in a recipe can be reduced, usually without noticeable difference in taste. One trick my wife uses when baking a cake is to substitute equal amounts of applesauce for the amount of oil called for. If the recipe calls for 1/3 cup of oil—1/3 cup of applesauce works just as well.

One great help in cooking is the large variety of foods that are sold prepackaged, frozen, or prepared in the deli section (such as roasted chicken). These products mean that not everything needs to be cooked from scratch. Prepared foods can be especially convenient for something like mashed potatoes. For me, it hardly seems worthwhile to cook and mash the few potatoes we will be eating. If you do a lot of this type of cooking, my only caution is to compare the calorie content for different brands. You might be surprised at how great the difference is between them. Of course, you will also want to consider which ones taste best.

SHOPPING

One of the most important, and frequently time-consuming, parts of a cook's job is shopping. Almost every diet book I've ever read cautions about shopping while hungry. This is good advice. I'm a fairly strongly motivated person, but a trip to the market when I haven't just eaten, or at least had a snack, can be like walking into a quicksand-laden swamp.

"Man, look at those doughnuts," I might think as I pass by. Ditto the sushi in the deli case, ditto the cans of cashews on sale. By then the little appetite I had when I came in is becoming a gnawing sensation as I pass half a dozen more appetite-increasing delights.

Finally, I end up at the section where the lunch meat is positioned next to the cheese I came in for. I grab the cheese, and look up. Oh, no, there are small sticks of pepperoni hanging right there. What the heck, I think, a few bites of one of them won't hurt too much. But you get the picture. A couple of bites never quite does it. Bet you've been there yourself.

As mentioned earlier, low-calorie cooking begins with low-calorie shopping. If you are not already very familiar with the difference in calories between various types of meat, you've got some studying to do. And, by all means, take your calorie book to the store with you. Pork ribs, for example, are high in calories and should be saved for special occasions.

What if you had to choose between wieners or chicken breast for your barbecue? If you chose wieners, you might want to get more familiar with what's in the calorie book. But that's only part of the problem. Round steak has far fewer calories than T-bone, for example. If you choose round steak, not only will it probably require a different way of cooking, it will also probably take longer to make it tender enough to eat. That's why my round steaks go in the Crock-Pot.

Once again, the types of meat you buy and the ways you prepare them depend totally on your preferred methods of cooking and eating. But you need to stay conscious of the calorie differences in how you cook, or prepare things for the table. Even a very low calorie dish can be ruined by what you put on it. Take broccoli, for example. It's a great dish—unless you dress it up with gobs of butter or a cheese sauce. Any good book on nutrition can help you with this if you are not already familiar with lower calorie ways of cooking.

LABELS

Everything you ever wanted to know—and more. That's what you can find on labels these days. But that's not a bad thing. It's a great thing, actually. And not only because reading the labels lets you keep on top of your RMR caloric limit. The nutritional part of the labels can give you good guidance to make sure your decreased food intake does not result in damaging your health by improper eating. Cooks, especially, need to be aware of keeping everything as nutritionally balanced as possible.

The U.S. Food and Drug Administration Nutrition Facts information is printed on most packaged foods. It tells you how many calories and how much fat, carbohydrates, sodium and other nutrients are available in one serving of food. Most packaged foods contain more than a single serving. The serving sizes that appear on food labels are based on the FDA-established lists of foods. . . . To see how many servings a package has, check the "servings per container" listed on its Nutrition Facts. . . .

When cooking for yourself, use measuring cups and spoons to measure your usual food portions and compare them to standard serving sizes from Nutrition Facts of packaged food products for a week or so. Put the suggested serving size that appears on the label on your plate before you start eating.[7]

EATING OUT

How about some more tips on eating out? "I'd like a half a rack of ribs, and two sides of coleslaw to go." The very day I was writing this, that is the order I placed at a local restaurant—believe it or not. Outrageous? Not at all. Four ounces of barbecue pork rib meat is around 510 calories. When my wife, Bobbie, and I split the order, we each get only two ounces of meat, which is only around 255 calories. Hardly diet-busting for our big meal of the day. Of course, the coleslaw has to be added to that.

A far more frequent favorite of ours is Subway. One nice thing about

Subway is that the calorie content of every food they serve is on a little card they have for you. Also, I'm more satisfied with the sub than half of a half rack of ribs.

For those rare times it's just got to be pizza, we order vegetarian. The last time we were at a family gathering the fare for the day included pizza, salad with rotelli, fresh fruit, and a number of different pies. I maintained my RMR limit by eating a cup of salad, a cup of fruit, one slice of pizza and no pie.

Bobbie and I have developed a trick to help control our portions when we are eating out. We will order one dinner from the menu, and ask for two plates. I was shocked to discover that this is such a common practice in restaurants now that the waiter or waitress doesn't even bat an eye. Finally, if all else fails, we ask, "Would you please bring us a doggie bag?"

I'm sure you have your own favorites when it comes to sub sand-wiches, seafood, or ribs. Just be sure you keep your RMR limit in mind as you make choices from the menu and you will find that though you may need to alter your choices a bit, no food is completely off limits.

FORBIDDEN FOODS

Let's consider traditionally forbidden foods on many diets. If, for example, you're on a macrobiotic diet, there is probably a whole list of things you used to eat that are now forbidden. This quote illustrates how confining such a diet can be. "Avoid unnatural foods. Eating any type of processed foods is strictly forbidden. . . . Processed foods have been altered from their natural state, often to give them a longer shelf life. Avoid any products in which the methods used for processing foods include canning, freezing, refrigeration or dehydration."[8]

But why go on? You get the picture. On hundreds of diets from the Cave Man diet to a vegetarian diet, there are forbidden foods. This is so prevalent that one article defines all diets as unhealthy when they involve "the conscious restriction of the amounts or kind of foods you're allowed to eat for the express purpose of losing weight. . . . If you count grams of fat, opt for high-protein foods while shunning carbs, rely on 'safe' foods, beat yourself up for eating 'bad' foods, consciously or unconsciously undereat (which can trigger overeating later), use diet soft drinks or coffee to quell your hunger"[9] that is unhealthy.

So here's the list of forbidden foods on the RMR diet: albatross wings, bat's brains, caterpillars, dog food, eel eggs, and anything else you can come up with that is disgusting or ridiculous to complete the alphabetical list started above. Obviously, nothing is actually prohibited, but I'm personally not sure that I'll ever eat escargo or frog's legs.

Let's get back to "moderation in all things." That's not always true. When it comes to certain foods "a minimum of these things," might be a more productive way to think. These foods include things like chocolate, or prepared foods like wieners, sausages, brats, and lunch meats. These foods are "calorie dense," and should be used minimally.

The term "calorie dense" is a key part of Robert Pritikin's Pritikin diet. The original Pritkin diet was established by Robert's father, but Robert has adjusted his father's diet to focus more on the types of foods one eats. "He claims the concern is not calories, but rather how dense they are in any given food. . . . Some foods have more calories packed in them, bite for bite and pound for pound. . . . If we eat foods with fewer calories per pound, we can fill up on these foods and still have the kind of calorie deficit that we need to lose weight."[10]

On the RMR diet, this does not mean such calorie-dense foods are forbidden. Especially if you really love them. Some of them even have good nutritional values.

While I'm not sure that the nutritional value of Italian sausage, for example, makes it ideal for any diet, I could hardly consider a spaghetti sauce without it as being really scrumptious. Using the idea of "a minimum of these things," I have definitely changed my eating habits with items such as sausage. I used to eat two sausages regularly with my spaghetti. Now I eat only half of one.

All of this brings us back to portion control. A pound of steamed broccoli spears is around 115 calories and is not really abusing portion control—especially if it is eaten as a snack. A pound of baked potato on the other hand is around 560 calories. It doesn't matter when you eat that, it's probably way too much. Thus, in controlling your portions the amount of calories per portion is critical.

So while nothing is forbidden, how much we eat of those calorie-dense foods needs to be closely monitored. Portion control is as much about the calories per portion as it is about the amount of food on your plate.

NOTES

1. "Food Portions—Recognize and Control Food Portions," About.com, http://arthritis.about.com/od/weight/ht/foodportions.htm.
2. "Win—Publication—Just Enough for You," http://www.win.niddk.nih.gov/publications/just_enough.htm.
3. "Tips for Estimating Serving Sizes," MyFoodDiary.com, http://myfooddiary.com/resources/estimating_serving_sizes.asp.
4. *Obesity Education Initiative Electronic Textbook*, www.nhlbi.nih.gov/guidelines/obesity/e_txtbk/appndx/ba2a.htm.
5. "How Your Grill Can Help Your Diet," www.emaxhealth.com/11/141.html.
6. "Cooking With Sugar Substitutes," About.com, http://homecooking.about.com/library/weekly/bℓ010598b.htm
7. "Win—Publication—Just Enough for You," http://www.win.niddk.nih.gov/publications/just_enough.htm.
8. "How to Avoid Forbidden Foods on a Macrobiotic Diet," www.ehow.com/how_2214481_avoid-forbidden-foods-macrobiotic-diet.html.
9. "Are All Diets Unhealthy?" About.com http://womenshealth.about.com/od/fitnessandhealth/a/exrunawayeating.htm.
10. "The Pritikin Principle: What It Is," WebMD, www.webmd.com/diet/pritkin-principle-what-it-is.

7

Psychology of Weight Loss

Psychology is not just a bunch of head stuff used by psychiatrists as you lie on their couches. Psychological principles can be very beneficial in helping you achieve life's endeavors.

THE GOAL APPROACH QUOTIENT

One of these psychological principles is called, the "Goal Approach Quotient." In plain English, the Goal Approach Quotient means that the closer you get to your goal, the more motivation you have to finish it. Have you ever noticed in a hundred yard dash, just before the runners hit the tape they speed up? That's a Goal Approach Quotient. If the closer we get to our goal, the more motivation we have, doesn't it make sense to have goals close enough to be within our reach?

That's why it works to divide up any long term goals into shorter time frames. For example: Goal, to burn fifty pounds of fat. Okay, but you can take advantage of the goal approach quotient by setting your first goal at burning the first ten pounds, the second could be to have burned a total of twenty-five.

Once you've lost those first ten pounds, how far we still have to go might cause us to think we haven't accomplished much. My wife felt ten pounds was no big deal at first, so I went and got a ten pound bag of sugar and handed it to her. "See how much less fat you now have to carry around? See how much lighter your body is?" Bobbie was amazed. And you might be as well, if you try it.

And this is not just a technique I show others. I do it myself. I first did this after I'd lost twenty five pounds. I was amazed. By the time I'd lost fifty pounds and picked up a bag of bird seed weighing that much, I had a far greater understanding of how much damage I'd done to my body in carrying that much fat around with every step I took all those years. Even now, whenever I lift something with any weight to it, I think to myself, "I've burned more fat than this weighs."

But, on the RMR Diet, there are many more things to accomplish before the fat starts burning off in significant amounts. If you look at everything covered in this book so far, it may seem an overwhelming task to get on the diet and stay on it. But the basics of it are truly simple and easy to accomplish. The rest of this book is meant to inform you why it works, and give tips on how to make it work better and more easily for you.

The Goal Approach Quotient should be used to help you get started on the RMR diet. Once you determine your RMR limit, decide on a few of the first things you want to accomplish. The next chapter will be about setting goals and how to achieve them. But the Goal Approach Quotient can give you strength throughout the entire process.

Your first goal can be to measure the amounts of food you are currently eating and the amount of calories they contain. You can set your own time frame by when you will have reached this measurement goal. The closer you get to becoming familiar with measurements and calculating calories, the more you will be motivated. Actually limiting yourself to your RMR limit could be your next goal.

In summary, to have the Goal Approach Quotient work for you, you have to have a goal. Goals you create that aren't really important to you just don't work. The more important your goal is to you, the more motivation and excitement you will get as you get closer to meeting it. The same is true for goals that will take too long to reach. Of course you'll get excited when you approach it, but that will be a long time from now.

Why would a goal of measuring and calculating calories be a big enough goal to get excited about it? Because once you've done that, you've conquered one of the tedious tasks that keep many people from going on a successful diet in the first place!

Habits

Yet another thing in our psyches that can help us greatly is our habits. Most of the time when we think about or discuss habits, we think of bad habits. But each one of us has literally hundreds of good habits that help us get through life without even thinking about them.

One example of such day-to-day habits is sitting down at a table when it's time to eat. We just do it. We don't even have to think about it, and usually, we're not even aware we've done it, the habit is so much a part of us. Putting toothpaste on our toothbrush when we're ready to brush our teeth, opening a door when we're ready to go in some place or leave it, and scratching our head when it itches are other examples. In fact much of what we do in life is just a habit.

This is true because habits do, in fact, control our behavior, and are ways of behaving we do not even have to think about. That's where psychology comes in. If you have a good habit you would like to get better at, or a bad habit you'd like to get rid of, there are little tricks you can do to make you more successful in changing your habits.

Since most literature is on breaking bad habits, let's look at that. One article says, "Regardless of the nature of the habits, the technique of habit reversal usually works very well in breaking them. . . . Recognize that the habit is a strong or persistent urge that is not rooted in deeper psychological problems."

This same article then outlines a number of techniques useful in kicking an old habit.

> Keep precise records of urges and count the number of times that you actually succumb to them. It has been shown that the very process of counting and record keeping tends to give one an immediate sense of control over the habit. . . .
>
> Learn relaxation methods as a means of combating the urges. . . . Substitute a response that is incompatible with the unwanted behavior. For example, brushing your teeth instead of eating a cookie. . . . If you really desire to quit the habit, this . . . process really works.[1]

Another article makes it even simpler by offering three tips for breaking bad habits. "Every single bad habit can be broken. . . . Here's how: The first step is to figure out when—and why . . . 'If you can notice when you're doing it and under what circumstances and what feelings are attached to it, you might be able to figure out why you are doing it and stop."

The second step is to, "Log it. . . this will help you establish a baseline . . . and what goes through your head. . . . This will make your bad habit more conscious." And the third step is to practice the, "Bait and Switch. Once you realize when and why you are . . . engaging in any bad habit, the next logical step is to find a not-quite-as annoying temporary or permanent replacement for it."[2]

The first thing is to notice about these articles is that they are talking about breaking very difficult habits like always reaching for food when you're unhappy or annoyed. Such harmful habits can break a diet and we will cover them in more detail later. Second, notice the similarities in the articles. Both talk about keeping a record—another good thing to put in your journal—and the technique called "Bait and Switch," which is shown in the first article with the line, "brushing your teeth instead of eating a cookie."

We will be making full use of these techniques for changing some simple, day-to-day habits of the way you eat now into habits that will support your RMR plan and make it more efficient in burning fat.

It is said it takes three weeks to either break an old habit or to create a new one. Depending on how minor or serious the habit is, it may be accomplished in a shorter time, or take a little longer. This process is called the "Three Week Habit Replacement Program."

Just one example of a habit that can be replaced and can become such a part of us that we no longer have to think about it is the habit of going into a gas station on the way to work each morning for a cream-filled doughnut. By incorporating the simple "Bait and Switch" of getting a piece of beef jerky instead, in three weeks or less, we'll be cutting our daily calorie intake by around 250 calories. Over five days per week, that's 1150, and for a month it would be 4600, or about a pound and a third of extra fat lost while still eating the same amount as you were eating before the switch.

Naturally, the many simple habit replacements you choose will not require that you log them into your journals unless the results you achieve are especially pleasing or the old habit was particularly hard to break. You can save the complete habit breaking program for more severe problems like impulsive eating.

It works best if you create one new habit at a time. "Yeah, yeah," you might think, "but if each one takes three weeks, I could be at this for months." So? What else will you be doing? It helps to remember that replacing a bad habit with a good one has a double pay off. Not only do you rid yourself of something that sabotaged you, you put in place a benefit that can serve you from now on.

PERSONAL MYTHS

But habits are not the only thing, psychologically, that control our eating. There are also eating superstitions, or if you prefer, myths. We can easily see that many superstitions from the past were actually myths. For example, the earth is the center of the universe, the sun circles the earth, and we must find and burn witches. At one time all of these were considered true.

When you allow your personal myths to become reality they use you and rarely for the better. When we thought there were witches, we burned people at the stake. It wasn't our inhumanity that caused us to do this, it was our myths.

To emphasize how your personal myth can use you, let's look at black cats. If I say black cats are bad luck, I now have to manage my exposure to black cats. But if instead I say, thinking black cats is bad luck is just a myth, that belief ceases to control my behavior.

Here's one of my personal myths: There is no diet that will help me lose weight and keep it off once it's lost. Besides, they're all a pain in the posterior, and too hard to follow. That's just the way it is.

If I say I just can't control my appetite and have to overeat at times, I have two strikes against me on any diet I might go on. If I say the fact that I can't control my eating at times although I'm not hungry is a myth, I am not controlled by that myth.

Before Columbus, everyone knew that if you sailed too far in one direction, you would fall of the edge of the world. That's just what the danger of sailing too far was. The way Columbus proved you wouldn't sail off the edge of the world was to sail to the Americas. The way you can prove your own myths are invalid is to contradict them by losing weight and keeping it off.

When it comes to losing weight, many of us have weight loss myths. If, so far, in your life you have tried to explain why you're overweight with a sentence that begins something like, "The reason I have a weight problem is . . ." you are probably talking about a myth. Some more examples of myths that use us are: I overeat because food is one of the most important things in my life. I overeat because family is important and we are always getting together over food. I overeat because we are poor and can only afford those cheap, high calorie things like beans, rice, and potatoes. I weigh more than I should because I'm big boned.

All of these, and many more, are inaccurate. The only reason you are overweight is that you eat more calories than your metabolism uses.

Often your personal myths are not your fault: they are founded on something you were once told and had no reason to disbelieve. For example, most of my life I was told that being fat was not only unhealthy, but that skinny people lived longer. Now they say the life expectancy of people in older age is increased if they are carrying a few extra pounds. So, in fact, a little extra fat may not only not kill you, it may help you to live longer.

Another myth I used to have is that to be truly healthy, vegetables need to be eaten raw. Not long ago I learned that vegetables do not need to be raw to be healthy. In fact some vegetables, such as carrots, are even healthier cooked. So if raw vegetables are not your favorite, cooked vegetables will serve as well when it comes to taming the snacking snake pit and getting good nutrition.

For years I was plagued by the myth that any food I ate late at night or just before going to bed would turn to fat during the night. One of the times when I am most in need of a snack is in the evening. This is true especially just before bedtime. Others may not have this problem, and some may have it worse than I do.

On past diets I would eat late in the evening and "know" I had ruined my diet for that day. Then, when I went off the diet, I would eat something at night and "know," once again, that this would make me fat. My myth controlled me.

This all reminds me of what my elderly step-mother once said. "First they tell you shouldn't do something, but should do something else. Then, in a few years, they say that is wrong, and you should do it. It makes you wonder, doesn't it? Does anybody really know what they're talking about out there?"

So what can you do about your personal myths? For starters, recognizing them can, by itself, help you get where you want to be. When you recognize them, you at least have the opportunity to decide whether you will continue to let them control you, or if you're going to control them. If you don't recognize them, name them as myths, and no longer let them use you, your chance of succeeding is probably nil.

So, how can you recognize them? Begin by logging all the reasons you think you overeat, or the excuses you give yourself when you eat into your journal. This can be extremely valuable for the same psychological reasons that were explained in the previous section about breaking bad habits. Plus, without keeping such a record what is going on can easily be lost.

The types of things you should be logging in are what you believe are the reasons you don't follow your RMR plan. Log in how often something causes a problem, how you feel about it, and how you feel about trying to change it. You should also log in why you are overeating and what you are eating at those times.

Once you recognize these myths or excuses and see what they are costing you, you will have the opportunity to do those things necessary to stop letting the myths or excuses use you. By keeping track you will also begin to see just how often these myths reoccur. The more you see how they are using you, the more incentive and power you will have to change them. This incentive and power can go a long way to achieving what you want without any further action on your part.

EMOTIONAL EATING

If you can't seem to change your personal myths, or you feel you just have no control over them, you have probably left the arena of myths and excuses and entered the arena of emotional eating. This is one of the biggest causes of all diet failures.

Emotional eating leading to overeating is a habit that can be taught unintentionally early on. It is the idea that food can be used to provide comfort or used as a reward. Many parents will take their children out for ice cream or junk food when they have had a bad day at school, whenever they had to get shots . . . or maybe just because the parent felt guilty over something done to the child. Also, parents may reward a child with food/junk food for good grades, good behavior, or for a bribery of sorts. . . .

Emotional eating/overeating in the young or the old can stem from boredom. Other factors that lead to emotional eating/overeating are: insecurities at a social event, stress, fatigue, tension, depression, anger, and loneliness.

The best way to combat emotional eating/overeating is to monitor your habits. If you find that you are overeating every time you and your significant other argue or you find that you are overeating every time your in-laws are in town then change your behavior. When you are staring into the refrigerator, drumming up a snack, and when you are not even hungry, stop and go outside and take a walk, read a book or magazine, do some laundry instead, call a friend and invite them to a movie, or go to one alone. Distracting yourself with something else that you enjoy is key to avoiding emotional eating and overeating.[3]

It might be useful to consider that some psychological principles are so effective that they can be used in many areas. Much of the above was covered in the discussion of the three week habit replacement program. In fact, the three basic steps: start logging your habits into a journal, being aware every time you're tempted, and the bait and switch method were all there.

Basically, there are only two types of emotional overeating. Either of them will become a diet buster if continued over time. The first is high calorie snacking: reaching for a candy bar, bowl of ice cream, or a bag of potato chips. The second is binge eating, which is when you begin eating until you've gone way over even normal meal quantities. I have, in the past, been plagued by both of these. Of the two, binge eating is by far the more serious.

The first thing to recognize when you find yourself doing either of these things is that you have not ruined anything. While we humans are very powerful in many ways, we sometimes "blow it" no matter what we are engaged in. If, however, you recognize the problem and start to change it, you are once again on the road to success. Obviously, it would be nice to change your emotional eating right away. But in your journal if you can at least notice that you have cut down the number of times you do it from every day to only four times a week, you will have proven two things. First, you do have some control over it. Second, you are already on the road to mastering it.

One article I found provided information to help you recognize binge eating. "Frequent episodes of uncontrollable binge eating; feeling extremely distressed or upset during or after bingeing; no regular attempts to 'make up' for the binges through vomiting, fasting, or over-exercising."[4]

If you vomit after you binge you are into bulimia, and if you fast too often you are into anorexia. Both of which are beyond the scope and purpose of this book and will need extra professional help.

The same article quoted above continues, offering more information and some tips on how to curb your binge eating.

The problem is that emotional eating doesn't solve anything. It may be comforting for a brief moment, but then reality sets back in, along with regret and self-loathing. . . . Unfortunately, weight gain only reinforces compulsive eating. It's not that people with binge eating disorder don't care about their bodies; they agonize over their ballooning weight. But the worse they feel about themselves and their appearance, the more they use food to cope. It becomes a vicious cycle: eating to feel better, feeling even worse, and then turning back to food for relief. . . .

You must develop a healthier relationship with food—a relationship that's based on meeting your nutritional needs, not your emotional ones. . . . Eating right and listening to your body is an essential step in stopping binge eating. Other strategies that help include practicing relaxation techniques, staying connected to family and friends, and making time for things you enjoy as part of your daily schedule.

Eat breakfast—skipping breakfast often leads to overeating later in the day.

Avoid temptation—you're much more likely to overeat if you have junk food, desserts, and unhealthy snacks in the house. Remove the temptation by clearing your fridge and cupboards of your favorite binge foods.

Exercise—not only will exercise help you lose weight in a healthy way, but it also lifts depression, improves overall health, and reduces stress. The natural mood-boosting effects of exercise can help put a stop to emotional eating.

Distress—learn how to cope with stress in healthy ways that don't involve food.[5]

UNCONSCIOUS EATING

There is one other psychological item that needs to be discussed here, and that is unconscious snacking or eating. Some of the information about this issue has already been covered, but more needs to be said.

If you're like me, it is not unusual to be in the fridge looking for something, and then reach for a piece of that baked ham, or some of that cheddar cheese, or anything else there that calls to me. Or if there is a can of nuts on the counter, I may take a handful as I pass by. I don't plan it; I don't think about it; I just eat it. This next article talks about that very thing.

Does your hand put food in your mouth without any conscious thought? Do you eat in front of your computer, television, or while on the phone? Do you have trouble recalling what exactly you ate? Then you might be an unconscious eater. Unconscious eaters eat mindlessly, paying little if any attention to what they eat; food is just one more multitasking item.

This type of eating can lead to a multitude of unwanted results, namely weight gain and poor food choices that leave you feeling sluggish. If you are trying to lose weight, then work on becoming more aware of what exactly you are eating by practicing mindful eating. Mindful eating allows you to be satisfied with less food and without fighting with yourself to stop eating.

To stop eating unconsciously stop multitasking when you eat. . . . Don't be watching TV or working. You need to be more aware of the food you are eating at all times, even when you are with a group of friends. When eating at a social event it is easy to overeat because your attention is elsewhere.[6]

One thing they didn't mention is a tremendous benefit I discovered when I really started paying attention to what I ate. That is I started savoring food much more—and I thought I already knew how to enjoy food! I learned to do this in two ways. The first was that when I snacked, I ate the snack slowly and in small bites. The second was that at a meal, I would only put one type of food in my mouth at a time. Yummy.

NOTES

1. "Kicking Your Old Habits: Breaking Bad Habits For Good," http://athealth. com/consumer/disorders/badhabits.html.
2. Chang, Louse, M.D. "3 Easy Steps to Breaking Bad Habits," WebMD, http://www.webmd.com/balance/features/3-easy-steps-to-breaking-bad-habits.
3. Overeating Is Caused By Emotional Eating 75% of the Time," http://www. vaxa.com/weight-loss-overeating.cfm.
4. Melinda Smith, M.A.; Suzanne Barston; Robert Segal, M.A; and Jeanne Segal, Ph.D.; "Binge Eating Disorder: Symptoms, Causes, Treatment, and Help," http://helpguide.org/mental/binge_eating_disorder.htm.
5. Ibid.
6. "Is Unconscious Eating Making You Fat?" http://ezinearticles.com/?Is-Unconscious-Eating-Making-You-Fat?&id=1060306.

8

Create a Plan

Any good plan is composed of a number of different parts that handle different problems and achieve desired outcomes. Your journal should start out with your plan.

Planning is such a vital part of the success of RMR that it would seem it should at least be in the second chapter, if not before. However, to create an effective plan, you must first have some knowledge about what you are planning for, why you are planning for that, and how each part of your plan will contribute to your success.

Before you start, remember: you are the one who determines if you will make a formal plan. If so, some things that you could include in your own plan are what you will do, what you will eat, and when you will eat. You could also consider how you will make the changes that come closest to fitting comfortably into who you are and what you like and don't like.

One thing that makes the RMR diet different from every other diet out there is that it teaches you more than just what to eat and what not to eat. In this chapter you will learn to create a personalized plan to help you begin, stay on, and eventually end your diet. If you're not into planning and recording, just read what follows and keep as much of it as you can in your mind. As with everything in the RMR diet, do it the way that works for you!

PLAN HOW YOU WILL KEEP YOUR RECORDS

As you think about how you will keep your records, consider the following.

> The next time you set out to lose weight, how would you like to double—or even triple—your weight loss? . . . This is the secret ingredient—record keeping. We realize that keeping track of what you eat and how much you exercise is just one more thing to add to an already busy day. But a study . . . found that weight loss increased from five pounds to triple that amount in participants who were the most conscientious about keeping a food diary.
>
> Scientists don't know exactly why keeping a record boosts weight-loss success, but another study of successful losers suggests that monitoring yourself on a daily basis helps you plan your meals and activity and allows you to track how well you performed against the plan. It may be that the process of keeping track makes you more mindful of the importance of the decisions you make each day.
>
> In addition to a food and activity diary, some people keep a journal. Weight loss can be challenging and you may find it helpful to record your feelings and concerns at the end of each day. It helps to include an affirmation in your journal entry. For example, "I am taking control of my weight to become healthier and more energetic." Select an affirmation that is meaningful to you, and concentrate on it as you go to sleep.[1]

PLAN YOUR GOALS

Setting goals is one of the most important parts of beginning any diet. Goals should be meaningful and important to you. The more important they are, the more motivated you will be to achieve them.

How you phrase your goals is also important. "I want to lose 65 pounds," is not a goal, necessarily, and focuses on the unpleasant process of having to lose 65 pounds. "I want to weigh 165, or 145, or 135 pounds," is a benchmark that focuses on the outcome, not the way of getting there. That is much more empowering. Other such goals are: I want a waist size of ___; I want my buttocks to be only___ inches; I want to wear ____ size dresses (or pants); and everything else you can think of that you want as a benefit from the RMR diet.

Plan some goal posts along the way

Once your end goals are decided upon, begin setting goal posts, or mile markers, or whatever else you choose to call them to divide up these larger goals. Set goal posts that are meaningful to you and that are not too far distant. Getting even one quarter of the way to where you want to end up can be very satisfying if that is a meaningful division of your end goal. The Goal Approach Quotient discussed in the last chapter emphasized how getting closer to a goal post can give you that extra boost.

Would a short term goal of losing five pounds be meaningful to you? If not, how about ten pounds? Would a goal of actually getting fully on the program within a month be meaningful? How about a goal of beginning to handle your chocolate or your binge eating within two weeks?

Plan your rewards

One important motivation is "to offer yourself a reward program. People need rewards in all aspects of life. For example, we go to work so we can get a reward—a paycheck. . . . This rewards style program should carry over into your diet. If you meet your exercise goal for the week, buy yourself that new album you've been reading reviews of. If you stay within your calorie limits, go see a movie on Saturday afternoon (just be sure to take some dried fruit or other healthy snack). Little rewards along the way will help keep you motivated." [4]

Psychologically, the sooner you can reward yourself after achieving a goal, the better it works. A quick small reward is more effective than a larger reward later.

One cardinal rule, however: your rewards cannot include food, with two exceptions. The first is that you can cook a meal you particularly enjoy—maybe something a little too expensive to eat often. The second is that you can go out to eat as a reward, as long as you don't overeat at the restaurant, of course.

Plan how you will measure your successes

The value of recording weight for motivation and being able to reward yourself has already been covered. Recording your weight can also help you determine what goal-post weights are best to allow the Goal Approach Quotient to work for you.

"How often should you weigh yourself? Many popular weight loss plans, such as Weight Watchers, do not recommend weighing yourself daily. Instead, they recommend stepping on the scales once per week, or even less frequently. Our weight fluctuates somewhat from day to day and daily weighing can lead to discouragement and potential sabotage if you see a higher number on the scale than you did on the day before."[5]

As I mentioned earlier, weighing should be done on the same day of the week, at the same time of day, and wearing the same amount of clothing. This will help to standardize and control as many of the variables that may show an inaccurate weight.

PLAN YOUR CALORIES

Once you know what the value of your RMR is, you can plan how many calories you will consume each day. Are you going to start with the RMR limit and see how it goes? Or are you going to cut that limit by a hundred or more (very few more) to get you off to a faster start?

Plan how you will determine your calories

First plan which references you will use to determine calories. If you don't have a good calorie book, get one.

As you know, you will also need measuring spoons, cups, and a small scale. Such measuring is sometimes tedious and having to measure every single little thing every time is ridiculous. Still, to learn what works in the types and amounts of food you eat, there is no better way. If you're missing something such as a scale, or enough different-sized measuring cups, get them.

Another important thing to consider as you plan is whether you cook just for yourself or for others. If you're cooking larger meals for others, make sure you plan how you will know the calories for the serving sizes you will eat for that meal.

Either way, part of this must include how you are going keep track of what is working and what is not, once your scale shows you. Keeping track is important so you can discover the value of any calorie changes you make. Are you losing weight faster? Slower? Or is the change making no difference at all?

Plan how you will record your calories

I keep my records on the Daily Calorie Record, but after a couple of months, I throw the old ones away. In truth, the records are far more useful at first than they are later on. At first, if I wanted to know how many calories that banana I ate was, I just looked back two days to see how what I recorded when I ate one the day before yesterday. Now I only need to do that when I eat a calorie-dense food for which I had to calculate the exact amount of calories it contained when I first cooked it.

As I neared my final weight, I even stopped recording or measuring and just estimated the values. However, after three weeks, I stopped burning fat. I realized that my portions were creeping up on me. I then began to make the type of change you will probably want to make as your experience with this diet grows: I only resumed measuring the quantity or weight of more calorie-dense foods such as cheese, pot roast, and nuts. I already knew the amount of calories for each amount.

When I was ready to shift from RMR to BMR, I was a little surprised that I had to start measuring and recording the day's totals again. Not so I wouldn't eat too much, but so I could eat more without going over my BMR limit.

PLAN YOUR MEALS

One thing it pays to look at is the times of day you will eat. The value of eating at the same time every day (when possible) has been stressed. If you do not normally eat meals at the same times, you might plan to do this more often.

> Why plan meals? The goal of meal planning is predictable and reliable daily calorie intake. . . . Planning meals in advance may seem foreign; an act that stamps out some of the precious spontaneity that makes life enjoyable. I think you'll see the reality isn't that bad, but first consider why planning meals is worth discussing at all . . . by trying to "wing it" with regard to what you eat, to balance your long term calorie intake meal by meal, making every decision on the spur of the moment, you're placing . . . your own health in the hands of a process you know inevitably leads to serious trouble.[6]

Here is another choice: "Make your eating plan automatic. . . . Eat the same thing for breakfast and lunch almost every day. Yes, every day. People who minimize food choices lose more weight."[7]

As with any advice I have given, or studies I have quoted, one size does not fit all. Don't let any part of this book discourage you or make it difficult to stay within your RMR limit. Personally, eating the same thing every day would become so boring and unrewarding to me, I'd give up for sure. But perhaps something like that would work for you. Whatever you do, plan your meals around foods you know and like. If you start cooking foods you don't normally eat, make sure you're not in the starvation mode.

Here is how I handled meal planning. My wife, Bobbie, and I share cooking. We do not even plan on which days, or for which meals one or the other of us will cook. Many things control this. For instance, one of us may ask the other, "How would you like some _____?" This is interpreted as, "I'd like to cook that, would it be all right with you?"

Then, when that person cooks, it behooves him or her to also know how much the servings are, and how many calories there are in a serving.

One difference between us is that she is allowed fewer calories on her RMR than I am. So, let's say she decides on a some roast beef we have left over in the fridge, and half a microwaved potato each. She will take the appropriate servings for her, and I might take more of the beef than she gets, or add an apple to get my calories up to where they should be.

Sometimes one or the other of us will ask, "What should we have for lunch?" If I feel like something, and she agrees, I'll usually cook it. If she suggests something else, she'll usually cook it. Once a week or so, neither of us will feel like cooking and we'll agree to go to Subway for a sandwich.

In short, and the following should not come as a surprise, plan your meals in the way that best suits you.

Plan how you will snack

The great importance of snacking on this diet has already been covered. So have the numerous choices of snacks that are available. One other thing I would recommend is that you visit your grocery store or a health food store to look over the variety of healthy, lower calorie snacks you might enjoy. Another thing that definitely needs planning are emergency snacks.

> It's 3 p.m. and you're craving something sweet . . . and something salty. Before you put your quarters into the closest vending machine, consider some healthy alternatives to potato chips and candy bars. . . . Emergency foods you want tend to be foods that are a little crunchy with some sweetness to them.
>
> Apples, carrots and nuts are great snacks to consider. A glass of vegetable juice also takes the edge off. . . . One snack you may not have thought of are breath strips. . . A lot of times, we have a craving center in our brain that says put something in me. . . . It doesn't tell you what.

Another way to fight fat is to spice it up! Adding red pepper flakes or cinnamon to your food can reduce your appetite. Starting with a smaller plate also helps you eat 33 percent less. [8]

Using a smaller plate has already been covered, but the fact that it can save you 33 percent was worth mentioning. In addition to the snacks you plan and take with you each day, you should have some packages of emergency snacks on hand for those times you have to go somewhere quickly and don't have time to put snacks into baggies. Knowing you have snacks available for emergencies reduces a lot of pressure when such occasions arise.

In addition to planning such things as how to keep higher calorie snacks out of sight, you should also plan how you will be able to enjoy potato chips, tortilla corn chips, saltines, nuts, raisins, chocolate bars, chocolate covered peanuts, and all the rest without eating a whole package. One thing is for sure: if you take the whole package somewhere with you, you're going to blow it.

In planning this part of snacking, plan just how many potato chips, chocolate, trail mix, nuts, and other such items you can safely eat. Then when you go for them, you will know exactly how much you should take—and exactly how much not to take!

One useful tool we have found effective is to keep a ¼ cup measuring cup inside a bag of nuts, for example. That way, when you're ready to snack, you don't have to get the appropriate measure. If not, measuring it may give way to, "Oh, I'll just take a handful."

Of all the parts of this RMR eating process, snacking is one of the most rewarding and satisfying.

Plan healthy shopping
Plan what you will do to keep from shopping when you are hungry. Plan what you'll do to learn which cuts of meat are high in fat and which are lower. Plan how you'll resist impulse buying of foods or snacks in a store that "call to you" while you're in the store. Plan how you'll resist the temptation to bring home things that contribute to emotional snacking, or to control how much of them you will bring home. Plan which foods you need to start buying more of in order to balance your food pyramid.

Plan how you will dine out
It is important to have a plan in place before you ever go through the doors of a buffet or restaurant. What are you capable of doing to maintain

your RMR limit? Can you do anything in advance to help insure that you won't?

As I began changing my eating habits on the RMR diet, I found there was one huge benefit, but unexpected benefit. Handling buffets had previously been big problem for me, but the first time I used my new technique of slowing down, I was amazed that one plate satisfied me. It took me longer to eat that plate than it did for the other people in my group to eat two or three plates. I'm reasonably certain I left feeling more satisfied than the others too.

PLAN HOW YOU WILL CHANGE YOUR HABITS

Imagine that you are on the diet. You're losing weight at a steady rate, you're not hungry all the time, and you no longer crave those huge amounts you used to eat. You're on your way and things are going great. But what would happen if you asked yourself what new habit you could create to supplement your eating plan for the rest of your life? One example is to change the rate at which you eat food. Again, the key here is recognition.

> When people eat more slowly, they eat less. In a study at the University of Rhode Island, 30 healthy weight women were asked to eat a pasta dish served with water until they were full.
>
> "When encouraged to eat quickly with a large spoon, they consumed 646 calories in about nine minutes. But another day when they had smaller spoons and were told to put their utensils down between bites and chew each mouthful between 15 and 20 times, they took an average of 579 calories in about 29 minutes. The women judged the more leisurely meal as more satisfying—even though they ate less.[9]

Interestingly, studies show that when we start eating, the brain releases chemicals to tell us, among many other things, when we have feelings of being full. Just one of these is serotonin, which "regulates sleep, reduces pain and appetite, and generally calms you down and improves your mood."[10]

Unfortunately, it takes time for the brain to release these chemicals. It is not instantaneous. What accounts for the women in the study above both consuming fewer calories and reporting the meal as more satisfying? The answer is the twenty-nine minutes it took them to eat, thus giving their brains time to start releasing the chemicals.

I began slowing my eating habits like the women in the study above. One thing I found is that, while the chemicals don't kick in immediately, it doesn't take anywhere near twenty-nine minutes. Twenty minutes seems more accurate. Also, it seemed to kick in even faster at different times, depending on what type of food I was eating.

Remembering that it takes three weeks to get the habit replacement technique in place, I exchanged my old way of eating for a new one. I used a smaller spoon (where appropriate) or did not put as much food on my fork as I had previously. I would put it down between bites. Instead of chewing the food in my mouth a specific number of times, I would simply swallow it when it was chewed sufficiently. Then I'd get another fork full and begin all over again.

In truth, laying the fork down and picking it up each time bugged me for some reason. I know that's probably the way people with "class" eat, but it was too foreign to my way of eating. I found that having to remember to put it down each time took away from my concentration on other things, like enjoying my food. The solution was simple, I'd just hold it and not put another bite in my mouth until my food was chewed and swallowed.

It took some concentration for over a week because I was so used to eating like a pig at a trough. Not only would I eat fast, but I would put a number of forks-full into my mouth while I was still chewing. But in concentrating, I discovered a couple of things that were important to me.

I would start watching for the feeling of being full to kick in—it never did. What did kick in was the feeling of being satisfied. Again, there is not a set time limit for this, so I had to start looking for it and become very familiar with what it felt like. Along with that feeling came the realization that feeling satisfied was more enjoyable than feeling full. I could, honestly, be more satisfied with less food than I ever had before. While this did not mean I would eat less during the day, it did mean I could snack more to make up for the smaller amount I was now eating during meals.

Finally, as I mentioned before, I began savoring food more than I had ever done before. Slowing my eating rate was important in helping me savor my food and making the RMR diet even more pleasant. Not only is the RMR diet more pleasant than any other diet I have been on before, but it is even more pleasant than the way I used to eat when I wasn't dieting.

Another thing you might put in your plans to change is taking a second helping after you've eaten as much as you should. This also involves letting those chemicals kick in. But some foods are so good, it really doesn't matter if I'm satisfied—I want more! The habit replacement I used for this one was to tell myself, "Okay, I'll have that second helping I want so badly, in a couple of minutes."

Then I'd get up and leave the table, and if I had to, even promise myself I'd come back and eat more in a few minutes. Then I'd replace that thought by doing something, such as starting to clean up the sink and load the dishwasher. I found at such times that it took only a little more time for my feelings of being satisfied to kick in strongly enough that I wouldn't go back for that second helping, even if part of me still wanted it. It is rare now for me to have to resort to this. Especially since I've slowed down my eating rate and adjusted my portion sizes significantly.

While it can take three weeks to create a new habit, reverting to an old one can happen quickly. One episode of overeating won't, necessarily, break your habit of eating smaller amounts. But eating a number of large portions in a short period of time can definitely make it necessary for you to have to begin creating the smaller portion habit again.

Plan how you will deal with emotional and unconscious eating

Since how to recognize emotional and unconscious eating and some of the ways to solve these problems has already been covered, what is important here is that you specifically and realistically plan how you are going to determine if either of these problems is getting in the way of your burning fat. It's not enough to say, "Oh, I know I've got that problem."

As mentioned, one of the keys to solving these problems is to recognize everything going on around them, such as your emotions when you eat. You can only get this valuable information if you have a plan to recognize and record in your journal every instance of when these problems occur.

Plan your exercise

In truth, you can lose weight without exercising at all. But it will take longer to get results. Not to mention you will miss out on the health benefits that come along with exercise. How you choose to exercise is not as important as that you choose to exercise.

PLAN HOW YOU WILL SHIFT FROM RMR TO BMR

How you will shift from RMR to BMR is, perhaps, the most important part of your diet to plan. As was mentioned in chapter one, you are now, and always will be, on a metabolic diet. How close your calorie intake matches your metabolism determines how much you weigh. The ultimate goal of the RMR diet is not simply to help you lose weight, but to help you enjoy a healthier, happier, more vigorous, and longer life.

Unless you know how you are going to shift to meeting your BMR, you really are missing the very most important part of this diet. Further, unless you plan for how you are going to make that change, after you've lost the weight you want, you will begin to gain it back. Plan to make this change slowly, over time.

The reason many diets fail is that they only concentrate on losing weight. They do not help dieters realize that those very things that make a diet so hard to get started on will creep back into their lives once they stop dieting.

Poor nutrition, portion creep, emotional eating, and other diet pitfalls will take longer to resurface once you get going on the RMR diet, but they will resurface unless you have a lifelong plan to keep them under control.

In conclusion, when making your plans think about those things about eating and being fat that make you unhappy with yourself, those things you presently do that are not appropriate on a diet, the things you presently do or feel that distress you while on a diet, some ways you could make your dieting experience easier or more satisfying, and anything else that would make your total success more certain.

NOTES

1. Shape Up America! Newsletter, 4/19/2008, www.shapeup.org/about/arch_news.nℓ0408.html.
2. "How to Keep Your Motivation High When You Are on a Diet," http://ezinearticles.com/?How-To-Keep-Your-Motivation-High-When-You-Are-On-A-Diet&id=489595.
3. "To Weigh, or Not to Weigh, That Is The Question" http://medicinenet.com/script
4. John Walker, "Planning Meals," http://www.fourmilab.ch/hackdiet/www.chapter1_3_2.html.
5. "*YOU: On a Diet* The 99-Second Version," www.realage.com/doctorcenter/articles.aspx?aid-10447.

6. "*YOU: On a Diet* Basics," www.oprah.com/slideshow/oprahshow/slideshow 2_ss_yourbody_20061102/4.

7. Christine M. Palumbo, "The Slow-Eating Diet" http://www.allure.com/magazine/2007/08/The_Slow_Eating_Diet.

8. "Serotonin" http://pages.prodigy.net/unohu/topics_sero.htm.

9

Time Lines
and Time

As I've said a number of times, the RMR diet is a lifelong thing. That's not bad news. The fantastic rewards like reaching the weight you've always dreamed of, improving your health, eating in a way that lets you enjoy all the foods you've come to love, and staying fit for the rest of your life make the RMR diet an appealing lifestyle even for those who don't need to lose weight. Once you establish the proper habits, that will just be the way you are and what you do. It will take far less thought and effort than your old way of eating. In short, it will become normal instead of feeling like a project.

How long this was going to take was one of my initial problems in going on the RMR plan. I didn't mind something that would last three months. I could stand it that long. But this? What I learned next didn't happen all at once, but came to me bit by bit, the longer I was on the RMR diet.

I came to feel this way of eating was not only the way I should have been eating all my life, but it was often downright enjoyable. Once I got started, the fact that I'd be involved over a long period of didn't seem bad at all. Especially when I learned I could even enjoy the trip.

In this chapter you will learn how to implement another planning and goal-setting tool, time lines. At first, your time lines will be just guesses. But as time passes you will become much more familiar with how long certain parts of the plan will take you. At first you may only get an idea how long one or two time lines will take. That's when you should adjust those time lines. By reviewing your time lines frequently, little by little you will be able to make more accurate predictions. At first you will find motivation as you begin seeing some of your time lines happening. Later, the motivation will come from the pride and satisfaction of having more of your time lines come to pass.

When I first began using this technique, it proved so useful I tried to achieve several time lines all at once. The only thing that changed was my great frustration when I completed hardly any of them in the time I was expecting.

At this point I said to myself, "Okay, let's forget the rest of it for two weeks and I'll achieve my time line of weighing the amount of meat I eat each day. It's a pain in the posterior, but at least it's moving me toward all I really want to accomplish."

When you get discouraged, look over your time lines, decide which ones are the most important, and then choose only one or two to get done right away.

Keep in mind that once you get going on this diet you will have reached a landmark that will improve almost everything with respect to your eating for the rest of your life. Since it is a lifetime thing, what would be so terrible about asking yourself, "Okay, I hate pinning myself down by trying to figure out when I'll have something done, but if it does help me achieve wonderful benefits, shouldn't I at least give time lines a try?"

SETTING YOUR OWN TIME LINES

There are many time lines along the way that you should both expect, use, and look forward to. Some are negative and may have plagued you before, but there is even help for these.

If you're losing one and a quarter pounds per week, it will take longer than if you're losing about two pounds, possibly a lot longer depending on how much weight you have to lose. So you must decide on a timeline that will work for you. Both of these goals are not only very achievable, but both are within a healthy rate of weight loss.

You can use these statistics to figure out about how long the RMR diet will take you. Once you know this, your other time lines can be estimated a little more accurately.

The first time line you should set is a time line for getting started. This refers to setting dates and perhaps recording them in your journal for when you will actually begin some of the goals you have set for yourself. For example, set a time line for when you will have everything in place to begin looking up calorie amounts, measuring, and recording your daily caloric intake.

Next, set a time line for when you will eat your meals during the day—if you can possibly plan this. Once you have begun, there are many more time lines you can set.

- Set a time line for when you will start controlling your portions of food.
- Set a time line for when you will actually limit yourself to your RMR calories.
- Set a time line for when you will know how to cook and portion meals according to your RMR goals.
- Set a time line for having your snacks adjusted to fully support the rest of your diet.
- Set a time line for when you will have adjusted what you eat to the Food Pyramid. Remember, good nutrition takes time.
- Set a time line for when your shopping will be done only when you are not hungry.
- Set a time line for when you will begin buying lower calorie, lower fat foods, and how you will resist impulse buying of foods that call to you.
- Set a time line for when you will have controlled your chocolate addiction, or similar cravings.
- Set a time line for when you will start making some of the other changes you might need to make to allow the program to be easier, more rewarding, and more enjoyable.
- Set a time line for when you will have lost the first five pounds.
- Set a time line for when you will review what you're doing, and change your time lines accordingly.
- Set a time line for when you will have lost the first ten pounds.
- Set a time line for when you will have lost the first twenty pounds.
- Set a time line for when you will be one quarter of the way to your final goal.
- Set a time line for when you will accomplish any other goals you might have.

There are, of course, more time lines to consider making. For example, I set a time line of one month for when people would begin to notice I'd lost weight. In truth, it took two months. Even then, not a lot of people noticed, and those who did were people who didn't see me often. Still, it's hard to explain the joy and satisfaction you feels when others begin to notice all you've done and how it's paying off.

You should also set a time line for when you will begin the BMR portion of the diet. At first this can only be estimated. But, as was mentioned in the discussion on goals, this is one of the most critical parts of the whole RMR, BMR way of life.

One way that works when deciding on this time line is to divide the amount of weight you need to lose by 1.5. That is roughly how many weeks it will take you. Naturally, you could divide by 2 (the maximum we should lose per week on average), but there are a number of reasons 1.5 works best. For example, as you get closer to your goal, your metabolism decreases and weight comes off slower than at first. My experience is that, after time, and as I got closer to my desired weight, how much I lost each week was no longer of much interest. As long as the general trend was still downward and I wasn't stuck on a plateau, I wasn't too concerned.

You should also set a time line for when you will review all your time lines and make adjustments. It pays to review your time lines often. When you do, you can make adjustments. For example, if you're not losing the pound or two per week that you can expect if you have a lot of weight to lose, you may need to look at your goals to see if any of them need tweaking.

Second, as you meet your guidelines and they begin to disappear, it is like looking at a road map of where you are, and how much further you have to go. Make no mistake, the more time lines you meet and the fewer you have left to accomplish, the more the Goal Approach Quotient will kick in.

DEALING WITH DISCOURAGEMENT

One potential problem with any diet is that you might get discouraged if you don't meet both your goals and time lines right away. Take heart. As long as you are practicing the four building blocks mentioned in Chapter One, you cannot fail. It may just take a little longer than you expected.

One article I found covers both periodic overeating and discouragement, "Forgive yourself. When you fall down and give in to your temptations don't beat yourself up for it. Forgive yourself and let it go immediately. Just start over again. No harm done. To criticize will only be self defeating. Don't let the weak moment become a reason to stay off the restrictions for a longer period of time or to give up. Just pick yourself up and begin again. Don't think of it as a failure, but rather a minor setback. Change happens slowly and usually involves many setbacks."[1]

Worrying about how long losing the weight will take can be very discouraging, especially if you have a lot of weight to lose. At least that's how I felt on most other diets. Even the thought of how long it was going to take when I started the RMR diet was so discouraging, I tried to put it out of my mind.

But this very discouragement will work to your benefit. First, because it will help the reality of what you are undertaking to set in. This is no easy thing. You are calling upon all that is strong in you, all that is determined within you, and all your hopes for a new and better life. Good for you! By focusing on these things, it helps you begin to understand just how powerful you really are, especially if being overweight has caused you to feel poorly about yourself.

Time lines are important because they can help you understand more fully that what you are undertaking is a lifelong thing. Unless you fully understand this, you will not be getting the full benefits of all you've given up, all you've done, and all your new life can be.

Burning the fat you want will take you six months, or a year, or in extreme cases two years—so what? On this plan we are looking at the rest of your life. And this little bit of time is hardly a blip on that time line.

A HISTORY OF DIETING

To help put your own dieting efforts in perspective, take a look at this time line of past diets. I found it fascinating.

1820 Vinegar and Water Diet. Made popular by Lord Byron.
1828 Low Carbohydrate Diet. First appeared in *The Physiology of Taste* by Jean Brilliat-Savarin.
1830 Graham's Diet. Only legacy: Invented Graham crackers.
1863 Banting's Low Carbohydrate Diet. "Banting" becomes a popular term for dieting.
1903 Horace Fletcher promotes "Fletcherizing." (Chewing food 32 times.)

1917 Calorie Counting. Introduced by Lulu Hunt Peters in her book *Diet and Health: With Key to the Calories.*

1925 Cigarette Diet. "Reach for a Lucky instead of a sweet."

1928 Inuit Meat-and-Fat Diet. Caribou, raw fish, and whale blubber.

1930 Hay Diet. Carbohydrates and proteins not allowed at same meal. Dr. Stoll's Diet Aid. First of the liquid diet drinks.

1934 Bananas and Skim Milk Diet. Backed by the United Fruit Company.

1950 Cabbage Soup Diet. Flatulence is listed as main side effect. Grapefruit Diet. Also known as the Hollywood Diet.

1960 Zen Macrobiotic Diet. Created by Japanese philosopher George Ohsawa.

1961 Calories Don't Count Diet. FDA filed charges regarding diet's claims.

1964 Drinking Man's Diet. Harvard School of Public Health declared diet unhealthful.

1970 Sleeping Beauty Diet. Individuals heavily sedated for several days. Liquid Protein Diets. Liquid protein drinks were low in vitamins and minerals.

1981 Beverly Hills Diet. Only fruit for first ten days but in unlimited amounts.

1985 Fit for Life. Avoid combining protein and carbohydrate foods. Caveman Diet. Foods from the Paleolithic Era.

1986 Rotation Diet. Rotating the number of calories taken from week to week.

1987 Scarsdale Diet. Low-carbohydrate, low-calorie diet plan.

1990 Cabbage Soup Diet. (Again)

1994 High Protein, Low Carb Diet. Dr. Atkin's version.

1995 Sugar Busters—Cut Sugar to Trim Fat. Eliminates refined carbohydrates.

1996 Eat Right for Your Type. Diet based on blood type.

1999 Juice, Fasting and Detoxification. Perennial dieting favorites reappear in combination.

2000 Raw Foods Diet. Focuses on uncooked, unprocessed organic foods.

2001 High Protein, Low Carb Diet. 1994 diet updated (by Dr. Atkins' son).

2004 Coconut Diet. Fats replaced with coconut oil.

2005 Cheater's Diet. Cheating on weekend is required.

2006 Maple Syrup Diet. Features a special syrup-lemon drink.[2]

NOTES

1. Cynthia Perkins, "10 Tips for Staying Within Your Dietary Restrictions," http://www.exmaxhealth.com/11/99.html.
2. Jennifer Starkey, "Fad Diet Timeline—Fad Diets Throughout the Years," http://www.eatright.org/cps/rde/xchg/ada/hs.xsl/media_11092_ENU_HTML.htm.

10

Motivation

One of the hardest parts of any weight loss program is staying motivated throughout it. Recent studies have shown that being able to maintain your motivation whilst trying to lose weight is absolutely critical in losing weight. In fact, some studies have suggested it is the essential success factor.

If you are like me, it is a lot easier to say you will stay motivated than to actually do it. There are always setbacks and bad days during the course of any diet. Learning how deal with those will help you tackle the tough times when you can feel your motivation slipping away.[1]

Many motivational techniques have already been discussed in this book. While not all of them have worked for me, many have and I suggest that they be recorded into your journal (or elsewhere) so they can be reviewed from time to time. Especially, when you start feeling a little down or depressed because something either isn't working or is hard to do.

In addition to those already discussed, this chapter will present a few more motivational techniques that will act as the icing on the cake. And don't worry, you can partake of all this icing. Not only will it not harm your RMR diet, but will be good for you.

On the RMR Diet I have achieved things that not only changed my life, but gave me great pleasure and increased motivation. One thing I have learned is the importance of rewarding yourself when you achieve a goal and being aware of the process of reaching your goals and recognizing them when they arrive.

Having experienced this process myself, and knowing how important those goals were once I got there, I began searching for a way to express their true value, and I came up with the word "landmark."

One of the dictionary definitions of a landmark is an event considered as a high point or a turning point. Far from being just another time when we reach a goal, and feel happy about it, a landmark is a permanent change that will benefit us for the rest of our lives. Because of this, achieving a landmark increases your comfort.

The Landmark of Comfort

Above all in life, we are driven to be comfortable. This is not laziness or a character flaw. It is a built-in mechanism to protect our lives. That which makes us uncomfortable is a sign, telling us that something is not right. Disharmony in our social lives makes us uncomfortable—a sign. Ill health makes us uncomfortable—a sign. Inability to be at ease with other people makes us uncomfortable—a sign.

But you get the picture. It is important for you to stay on the lookout for events and emotions that cause you to be uncomfortable and possibly to overeat. But it is equally vital that you notice which events and emotions are working for you and giving you pleasure or comfort.

What has comfort to do with burning fat? Everything. Your comfort in life influences what you eat, where you eat, with whom you eat, and how you celebrate. Any fat burning program that plunges you into discomfort is, eventually, bound to fail. You will only be able to take it for so long.

Equally as dangerous as the discomfort of being on a non-sustainable diet are periods when other things aside from your eating might be making you miserable. By watching out for these things that bring discomfort into your life, you have a far better chance of remaining focused on those important things that will put comfort back into our lives.

Discomfort can permeate every part of your life. Unhealthiness in your body causes both pain and illness, draining your ability to do things. How you look at yourself and how others view you can cause discomfort. To say being fat makes us uncomfortable is a considerable understatement. It almost drives some of us nuts. It affects not only the way we relate to ourselves, but how we relate to others and to our world. Ironically, one of the things that will give you comfort and help in how you relate to others is the actual burning of fat off your body. As the fat disappears, so will your discomfort.

This landmark of comfort can't be measured, nor can you set a time line for it to occur because there are so many variables involved in its occurrence. As you stay within your RMR limit, the fat will begin to disappear; as some of the effort you used to exert decreases, your vitality will increase. Then, one day, maybe without a particular event or reason, you will suddenly notice you are more comfortable. More comfortable in what you do; more comfortable around other people; and more comfortable with yourself—you have achieved the landmark of comfort, which will last a lifetime.

The Landmark of Appropriate Comfort Foods

At times, when things upset you or bug you, nothing may be needed more than a little comfort food. Without question, certain foods can give you a physical and psychological lift.

Comfort foods trigger the release of both endorphins and a related chemical called dopamine. You also get a quick surge of energy as the sugar or starch in some comfort foods hits your bloodstream. They are an important path toward this landmark of comfort.

This landmark will be achieved when you realize that comfort foods are no longer a thing to resist, or be ashamed of, but something you can enjoy and that contribute to all you are doing. As long as the quantity is controlled, comfort foods can continue to provide comfort and enjoyment the rest of your life.

The Landmark of Head-to-toe Health

When we think of burning fat, we mostly think about how good we'll look or how much smaller our clothes will be. The goals we set are mostly focused on what the scale will show and how long it will take us to get there.

There's nothing wrong with that, except that it is putting the cart before the horse. The greatest and most far-reaching effect is one undisputed fact: Properly done, the RMR diet will improve your health and vitality from head to toe.

To call this a landmark is neither an exaggeration nor a stretch of the imagination. Throughout my life I have studied nutrition, the advantages of being active, and the dangers of being overweight. So, when I went on the RMR diet, I really didn't give much thought to any of these things.

What I concentrated on were things like portion control, keeping a reasonably accurate count of calories, and many of the other things this book has discussed so far.

By the time I'd dropped fifty pounds, I suddenly realized that I had experienced this landmark of head-to-toe health. Everything about me from head to toe had changed. I hadn't expected it. I didn't plan for it. But suddenly I realized that my body would now be different for the rest of my life.

Just one example of this change was the disappearance of the pains in my joints, which I mentioned previously. Additionally, my clothes were not only a lot smaller, but I looked better in them and they fit better. I could get in and out of a car easier. From head to toe I was healthier, and the amount of energy I had literally blew me away. Now, I get so much more done in a day that you'd have to know me very well to even begin to believe it—especially given that I was never a couch potato to start with. Add to that my age, and, well, what more can I say? Is it any wonder I'm doing all I can to share this with you?

Until you experience it yourself, you really won't be able to appreciate this landmark. But when it does occur for you, you will have a far greater understanding and appreciation of what I mean by landmarks. You will know for certain how great a change you have made, how much better off you will be physically throughout life, and how much more comfort and enjoyment you will continue to experience.

The Landmark of Good Nutrition

You can actually damage yourself if you do not adhere strictly to certain nutritional rules. Everybody knows that. I learned how serious that damage can be back in 1959.

An overweight friend of mine tried to get me interested in the latest diet craze at the time. Since it involved eating only grapefruit, I wasn't really interested.[2] But by the time he'd lost thirty pounds and was really starting to look good, I decided to give it a try.

For me, that diet lasted less than a week. It ended when I learned that my friend had developed chest pains over the weekend and had gone to the doctor early Monday morning. The doctor never had the chance to examine him. He died of a heart attack sitting in the doctor's office, waiting to be seen. The doctor's guess was that he had been on this strange diet so long, he'd deprived his body of the essential nutrients necessary for good health.

Just think of how many young bulimic and anorexic people have died before doctors could reverse the damage done to their bodies. Not getting the proper nutrition is just part of the problem. Putting yourself into starvation mode makes it impossible to eat enough to even sustain the health you have now, let alone enhance it.

All the health risks of improper nutrition and being overweight would fill many volumes, but it is not the purpose here to cover too much of that. What I do want to focus on is that as you make your RMR program both a fat-burning program and a healthy eating plan, one day you will notice that your comfort, health, and vitality have all increased dramatically. And you will then realize that it is the healthy way you've been eating that is contributing just as much as your fat loss is. When this happens you will have achieved the landmark of good nutrition.

The Landmark of Freedom from Fear

If there's anything I hate in a diet program, a political program, an advertisement, or anything else of the same ilk, it is someone trying to scare me into something. Even if the things they are talking about are, in fact, pretty scary. I resent them bringing it up because in the past my best way of handling those fears was to try to forget about them.

Since the media is constantly talking about the dangers of obesity, we can't forget our fears for very long. We aren't allowed to forget about the troubles we are causing ourselves or what the future may bring.

Heart disease and stroke probably head the list of fears, but diabetes should run a close second. The first two can kill us, but diabetes can go a long way toward crippling both our way of life and our enjoyment of it, even if it doesn't kill us. Other things we should be afraid of are the types of cancer related to poor nutrition, kidney failure, and problems with our urinary tracts.

As you become successful at losing weight on the RMR diet, one day, if you stay in touch with what you are feeling and what is happening to you, you will suddenly notice that you are no longer afraid of what your excess fat and improper nutrition will do to your life. This is a true landmark in both comfort and enjoyment, and like the other landmarks we've discussed, this one will stay with you for as long as you live.

The Landmark of Not Grabbing for Food

One day you will notice you don't even think about grabbing for food. Can you even imagine how this will affect the rest of your life? Instead of constantly reaching for sweets like chocolate, items laden with fat such as cheese, pizza, and potato chips; or starchy foods like pasta, bread, and potatoes, you will eat at meals, and snack only when it is appropriate, and then on snacks you have trained yourself to eat.

This landmark will come when you have trained yourself to stay conscious of what you eat. To help this consciousness to occur, ask yourself questions like: Where am I when I reach for comfort food? Am I most tempted while shopping? How well does it work to keep certain goodies from lying in the kitchen? When I pass by the buffet do I grab for "just a little"? Again, this is highly individual process, but being conscious of your own urges is vital.

Keep in mind that we all have our own tastes and preferences when it comes to food. Since I was raised in a small coal mining community with many nationalities, I learned to enjoy an amazing variety of foods when eating at my friends' houses. Later, as I traveled to many places in the world, I would always partake of the favorite food of each culture. I reasoned that if millions of people ate and enjoyed a particular food, I would be missing out if I didn't learn to enjoy it also. I hate missing out on anything, so my rule became, "Try it, at least once."

Some of this food was so unusual at first, that I had to amend my rule of just trying it once. One example of such a peculiar food was sashimi (raw fish) in Japan. My new rule became, "I will try anything—twice." "After all," I reasoned, "it may be such a strange taste sensation the first time that I can't really tell whether I like it or not. The second time, I'll already be familiar with it and can better focus on whether or not it is something I'd like to eat again."

Another interesting point is that as I mentioned earlier, men and women frequently have different comfort foods. Unlike men, women don't generally have someone else placing hot food on the table for them, so foods that take a long time and a lot of effort to prepare are hardly comforting; a woman's comfort food is usually something she can just grab without all the work.

Thus, while this landmark is for both men and women, women will have both a harder time achieving it and find more satisfaction when it arrives.

The Landmark of Eliminating Your Emotional Eating

In the past, your moods affected the different types of foods you ate, the times you ate when you shouldn't have, and how much you ate (or overate). Because of that, eliminating your emotional eating is one of those landmarks that, by itself, could have prevented you from having to diet in the first place. More important, however, once it is achieved, this landmark can, by itself, be extremely valuable in creating a new lifestyle that never includes another diet as long as you live.

When you achieve this landmark it will revolutionize your eating for the rest of your life. It should be worked for, expected, and finally achieved. When you reach it, the only emotion that will accompany your eating will be the satisfaction from the food, and the satisfaction of knowing you are eating right.

The Landmark of Joy in Eating Out

When I weighed between two hundred fifty and three hundred pounds, dining out created problems for me. While I wasn't on a diet, I was self-conscious and frequently did not eat as much as I wanted to because I didn't want people to think I was a glutton. One look at me, and they already knew that, but I didn't want to reinforce it.

Then, when I would go on a diet, going to a restaurant was totally self-defeating. Before the RMR diet there was just no way I could not overeat. I'd hate myself for it, beat myself up, and as often as not decide that if I could no longer go out to eat, dieting just wasn't worth it.

Then, one day, after having been on the RMR diet for awhile, I realized that going to a restaurant was not only not a problem, but I looked forward to it and found joy and companionship with others during the meal. What a change! Again, it wasn't something I planned for, nor for that matter was I even aware such a change could take place—but it did.

The Landmark of Respect from Others

While I was eagerly awaiting the day when others would notice I was losing lots of weight, I was unprepared for the respect I was shown in the questions I was asked, the comments that were made, and the tone of voice in which all this was done. It was a little puzzling.

Then, it hit me like a brick thrown at my head. Whether or not they are fit themselves, all people know how hard it is to burn fat and are truly impressed by the few people they see doing it. And this respect only seemed to increase when they saw that I was keeping it off.

To say this landmark is life changing doesn't even come close.

LANDMARKS

So, what does all this have to do with motivation? Consider that if you get on the RMR diet, and stay on it until it's time to switch to your BMR limit, it will change your life in ways you had not even dreamed of previously. Every one of these changes brings joy, freedom from fear, great personal satisfaction, a new and better way to relate to yourself and the world, and great improvement in your health.

You may have thought you were well motivated because, for one thing, you've obtained a copy of this book and you've read it to this point. That's true. What is being said now not only does not take away from that, but it should help you to understand that you are truly motivated. You have what it takes to succeed. Now all that is left is to prove it to yourself and others.

When you first started reading, you knew what was motivating you to lose weight. But, by considering the landmarks, you should now also know that the rewards will be far greater than you ever imagined when you first picked up this book.

More important than what you know is everything you will experience as you meet each of these landmarks. Perhaps you wonder if you will really experience them, but one of the keys to changing that doubt will be the first time you achieve one. Once you experience that, your tentative faith that all the other landmarks will occur will change to eager anticipation. Again, now that you know these landmarks exist, be aware of the possibilities. Know what the landmarks are and watch for them. It will be well worth it.

As mentioned earlier, I never even knew they existed until they started happening because I never experienced them on any other diet I tried. But as each one occurred I became more and more aware that the RMR diet was not only superior to any of the others I had tried, but that it would also transform the lives of everyone who went on it and stayed on it.

So, finally, we get back to answering the question of what this has to do with motivation. I fully expect that the evidence that this diet can and will help you achieve your dreams will provide considerable motivation.

VISUALIZATION

Another valuable type of motivation is visualization.

They say a picture's worth a thousand words. . . . Dieting and weight loss require a lot of behavior changes, they require a lot of work. . . . In order to remain motivated enough to modify bad habits and maintain better ones, people often need more than sensible dieting and exercise programs, good intentions, and good support. They need to visualize successful results and believe that they're capable of changing. "Visualization techniques are very, very important both for dieting on a small scale and on a large scale. . . . When you have a picture of what you're trying to achieve, it helps you move in that direction. It tells you the track you want to be on and how you're going to get there."[3]

This extremely valuable technique is also emphasized in another article. "Building and shaping one's imagination can offer incredible results. . . . Rather than focus on nothing, focus on something. . . . Our imaginations have the ability to run wild, naturally, but also offer incredible ability . . . through simple visualization techniques and methods."[4] If being stressed is one of your problems, other techniques this article mentions as helpful include exercise, music, and meditation.

Related to the Landmark of Joy in Eating Out is a visualization that might be worth considering: "One of my motivations is to get down to a normal size, to walk in the mall and get lost in the crowd."[5]

Many people have trouble visualizing themselves, even when standing in front of a full-length mirror. The problem is that you see yourself every day, and since change happens slowly, you are not always truly aware of how much change has actually taken place.

I became aware of the following marvel of motivation when I was on a cruise to Alaska. One of the people with us took a picture of Bobbie and me. At that point I had barely lost half the weight I needed to lose. But when comparing that picture to one where I was still obese—I couldn't believe the change. If feasible for you, I suggest you have snapshots of yourself taken along the way on your own cruise to a thinner you.

NOTES

1. Paul Duxbury, "*How To Keep Your Motivation High When You Are On a Diet,*" http://ezinearticles.com/?How-To-Keep-Your-Motivation-High-When-You-Are-On-A-Diet&id=48959.
2. Jennifer Starkey, "Fad Diet Timeline—Fad Diets Throughout the Years," Grapefruit Hollywood Diet, http://www.eatright.org/cps/rde/xchg/ada/hs.xsl/media_11092_ENU_HTML.htm.
3. "Positive Image" www.dietdetective.com/content/view495/50/

---

4. KevinD, "Simple Things You Can Do to Reduce Stress," http://www.gather.com/viewArticle.jsp?articleId=281474977306067.

5. Sirlarry, "Do You Get Bigger When You Leave the House?" http://forum.lowcarber.org/archive/index.php/t-281197.html.

11

Enjoying
the RMR Diet

As was the case with motivation, many tips and tricks for enjoying the RMR diet and eating less have already been covered. Some others are worth considering, and a couple of them need to be reviewed in greater depth.

Diet Buddies

An important tip for both dieting and exercise that needs to be expanded is finding a friend or support group to become involved with. They need not even be on the same diet or exercise program as you. What works best is if they are people you can talk with and with whom you can share both your problems and successes. Naturally, if you're both doing the same thing, that is even more effective.

One article said, "Call a friend. If you can get a buddy system going this can be very helpful. Call your friend during times of weakness and talk it out. Make arrangements with your friend ahead of time and have a plan of action. Have your friend remind you of your goals or how badly you will feel after you [break] them. Have specific phrases for your friend to repeat back to you."[1]

The term "diet buddy" is used a lot, and the benefits of having one far outweigh the difficulty of finding one, even if you are the type of person who dislikes "group activities." Next best thing to having a buddy is finding a support group. A call to your local county health department, the YMCA, the YWCA, a hospital, or the health department in a nearby university might help you find one. As this next article shows, support can come from a variety of sources.

An exercise buddy who motivates you to show up for an early-morning walk . . . a neighbor who can watch your kids while you go for a run . . . a coworker who's also dieting to share healthy brown bag lunches with. These are just some of the many sources of support you'll need to call on as you take your weight-loss journey. . . . Take a few minutes to think about the kind of support you need as you face various weight-loss challenges—and how you'll get it. With a support game plan in hand, you're ready for just about anything.[2]

Before you read the following study, it would help to keep in mind that it covers many things about buddies. It is written by professionals who want to cover everything, and then some. If most of us gave even half the attention to choosing a marriage partner as this article recommends giving to choosing a diet buddy, divorce rates would plummet. So, don't let it make you think choosing a buddy is a tough and involved thing. Just keep in mind those parts of the article that would be useful to you.

There's no getting around it, the road to weight loss can be a bumpy one. But much like life's other journeys, the going can be smoother when you have someone to share it with.

That's where a diet buddy comes in—a partner who not only shares your weight loss and workout goals, but it can help you navigate a kinder, gentler path to sveltsville. Many experts now say buddying up can make the difference between failure and success with any weight loss plan. "Most people put all their effort into finding the right diet or exercise program but don't put any energy into creating a support and accountability system . . ." says Adam Shaffren, D.C. an exercise physiologist and chiropractor who is the author of *You Can't Lose Weight Alone.*

People fail not necessarily because they're following a bad weight loss plan, but because they lack a good support system. "It can be the deciding factor that makes a diet work—or not work."

What makes a good buddy? Most of us know what turns us on in a partner, and it's easy to count the virtues of our best friends. But if you're thinking of using these same guidelines to find a diet buddy, you could be making a mistake. . . .

Experts say that sometimes you would never tolerate a partner—like holding you accountable for every bite you take—could be the very qualities you need in a weight loss buddy.

Choosing a diet partner, like choosing as diet is a very personal matter . . . Just as there is no one diet that's perfect for every person, there is no one type of diet buddy that is universally better than another.

So how do you figure out what you need? Look deep inside yourself and be brutally honest about what you need to get your weight loss mojo working. Don't just focus on doing things together. Diet buddies are just two people who share a common goal and know they can count on each other to help them achieve that goal in whatever way it takes to do that.

For some that may mean working out together or getting together to cook or swap a couple times a week. For others, it can mean taking turns babysitting so that each of you can get to the gym separately. Another consideration is mutual availability. Both partners should agree up front on how much time and energy they have to devote to the partnership, and discuss what they need from each other during that time.

Also important: The primary mode of contact and support. If you're constantly monitoring your email and need a buddy who's always there when you send out the Instant Message S.O.S., be sure you pick a buddy who is as computer accessible as you. If what you really need is face-to-face contact, pick a buddy who has a similar need—and the time to share.

For some people, the anonymity of having an Internet buddy is the best solution. For others, it has to be someone who they can get together with for Wednesday night weigh in. It doesn't matter as long as both buddies want the same thing. No matter what your mode of communication, it's important that buddies spend time listening to each other. . . .

It's also important to recognize that encouragement comes in many different forms. For some people, it means hearing kind words, for others it means having someone come bay and literally drag them out of the house. . . . As long a both buddies know what the other needs and expects, then they can be there for each other.[3]

Whew! That's a lot to think about! This next article is strictly for women.

Man can feel perfectly comfortable choosing a woman as a weight loss buddy . . . if she will have him. A woman cannot diet with man because he thinks that weight loss is all about willpower. They decide to eat less and they do. They do not hear the cake calling their names. They do not see the cookies taunting them. . .

A woman cannot diet with a man because men have more muscle

mass. Therefore, they burn off fat faster than women burn fat. . . . A woman cannot diet with a man because men do not get PMS, or at least they will never admit it. Therefore, cravings and bloating do not slow down their progress.

A woman cannot diet with a man because watching the weight fall off a man is bad for a woman's self esteem. Men seem to lose weight almost miraculously. It is as if they will it to happen. Women do not have it that easy. If a woman were to measure her weight loss against her male study buddy, she would surely become depressed and give up.

A woman cannot diet with a man because no one will notice your twenty pound weight loss with him flaunting his 30-pound weight loss. It will make your success seem insignificant. A woman cannot diet with a man because men are sore losers. They are poor winners, too. They will sulk if you do lose weight faster, and they will taunt you if they lose weight faster.

Of course, if that man is your husband, you may not have a choice. If you are stuck dieting with a man, try comparing weight loss percentage, or BMI lost instead of pounds. It will help you feel better when the weight is falling off him. However, remember his muscles are heavier than your fat, so you have a better chance of winning the weight loss race if you truly compare apples to apples.[4]

I tried to get Bobbie to write a paragraph for me explaining how I wasn't anywhere near as bad as that as her diet buddy. She refused. She said that if I thought that, I was too delusional to be writing a book in the first place.

Here comes the last word on diet buddies. It's my all-time favorite.

Pets and owners in weight-loss study shed extra pounds faster than solo dieters. . . . People looking for a way to lose weight may want to trade in pills for a pooch. A first-of-its-king experiment to put people and their pets on a diet and exercise program found that both lost weight and kept it off, though dogs did better than their owners and didn't drive them crazy asking for food.

With two-thirds of Americans and one-fourth of pets overweight or obese, there's huge potential for this novel buddy system, experts say. "If you're looking for motivation and social support to lose weight, you probably don't have to look any further than the pet in your own home," said Dr. Robert Kushner of Northwestern Medical School in Chicago, who led the study.

Despite it's cuteness factor, the research actually was a big hairy deal, said Kushner who has done obesity studies for 20 years. . . . He and Kimberly Rudloff, a Chicago veterinarian enrolled three groups: 56 people, 53 dogs, and 36 dogs and their owners. . . . All were followed for one year.[5]

Previously, I gave tips on how you might find a support group.[6] Whether you do it online, with your spouse, a friend, or your pet, find someone who will motivate you to achieve your goals.

There was one other tip I learned at the time management workshop that is worth discussing. We all have problems remembering to do things we want or need to do. For example, say that you intended to put Swiss cheese on your shopping list, but you left the list in another room. Then your dog began chewing up your slipper, and—forget the list. You've probably had hundreds of such instances.

The tip to remedy this situation is simply to put something you can't miss out of place the moment you realize there will be a delay in accomplishing something you want to do. This tip is especially useful to me when I think of something just as I'm going to bed that I really want or need to do in the morning.

When that happens I do something like turn my clock radio sideways. Or, perhaps, put my wallet on top of the radio. When I wake up and see my wallet on top of my radio, covering the switch that turns the alarm off—bingo—I know that means I've got to ____.

When I first tried to slow my rate of eating, my old habit was such a part of me, that at the next meal, I would just grab a fork and start in. To help me remember, I decided to lay the small pepper shaker on its side at the end of every meal.

It didn't work. I forgot another rule: tell others in the family when you're going to do something weird like this, or when you'll need their help with something. Unfortunately, the next time I went to the table and was expecting to see the pepper shaker on its side, there it was, standing upright in all its glory.

"Bobbie, honey," I said, "I'm on one of those three week things. I'm using the pepper shaker to remind me." She knew what it was all about. Fortunately, after about a week I started remembering it every meal on my own. Once more our table looked normal with both the salt and pepper shakers upright.

CELEBRATIONS

Many people find that after they've been on the RMR program for awhile, it almost becomes second nature. They are comfortable with what they are doing and are satisfied with the results. But now comes the fun part of our new lifestyle. I call it fun and games because that's the feeling I have when I get to celebrate.

One way to celebrate is to invite others over and have a special meal. "How would you guys like some spaghetti?" That was the question I asked Norm and Beth, the older couple we eat out with every Friday. Beth already knew about my spaghetti before she ever married Norm, so their answer was just as I expected. Not only did we have fun during the meal, I enjoyed that sausage more than I can say. (Okay, okay, I enjoyed that half a sausage more than I can say.)

I invited my family over for a Dutch oven cookout the first fall I was on the RMR diet. This brings up some other possibilities anytime you're entertaining. One is to cook in some way in which you don't normally cook. One more fun change is to eat someplace other than your normal eating place. On a cool summer evening, the back porch is just one possibility. Out on the lawn on that round table with the umbrella over it is another.

For any celebration, whether with guests or without, it's always fun to decorate the dining area, even if it's just the kitchen table. Candles and flowers are common, and are often seen in movies to set up a romantic scene. Sometimes, movies even show those big tables with an important group of rich people, surrounded by ornate decorations, being waited on by one or more servants.

The choices for fun decorations are limited only by your own imagination. One Halloween dinner, for example, I included a scarecrow and pumpkins. We had so much fun, the scarecrow is now a member of the family. He lives on our shaded back porch where we keep our swing. Just looking at him reminds me that the RMR diet can be enjoyable.

Eating in a different place, cooking in a different way, or preparing a different food can be done anytime you eat, not just when you're entertaining. There are always those meals you save for special occasions, but on the RMR diet you can cook one of them as a reward for achieving almost any goal.

Another way to celebrate reaching a goal is to serve a meal in a much more elegant way than usual. We generally save Bobbie's prized Noritake

China for special occasions, but we have found it fun to use it for a special meal in order to make reaching a particularly important goal a very special occasion.

You can spice up your work lunches too. I don't do anything for fun at lunch when I'm substitute teaching because I teach in dozens of schools and I don't spend enough time in any one to get to know the other teachers. However, if you work at the same place—and like your coworkers—a little imagination can create fun times there as well.

NOTES

1. "10 Tips for Staying Within Your Dietary Restrictions," http://www. emaxhealth.com/11/99.html.
2. "Getting Support" http://www.eatingwell.com/diet/getting-support/ getting-support.html.
3. Colette Bouchez, "Choosing A Weight Loss Buddy," http://www. medicinenet.com/script/main/art.asp?articlekey=63993.
4. A. Hermitt, "Why Women Should Not Choose Men as Diet Buddies" http://associatedcontent.com/article/383811/why_women_should_not_ choose_men_as.html?cat=51.
5. "Dogs Make Good Diet Buddies," msnbc.com, http://www.msnbc.msn. com/id/65063787/.
6. One of the articles mentioned Internet buddies. If you'd like to try that, here are a couple of online dieting communities you could look into. http:// www.Oprah.com/Community and www.mydietbuddy.com. Of course, you should always use appropriate precautions when making friends online.

12

Working With Biology

Factors that Influence Obesity

It is unusual for families to have only one member with a weight problem. This fact points to the genetic causes behind weight gain. But, as with almost everything else concerning the rising obesity rate in our nation, genetics seems to be only one of a number of different causes.

Recent studies show a definite relationship between obesity in some people and their genes. "Science shows that genetics plays a role in becoming overweight or obese. Genes can directly cause obesity in disorders such as Bardet-Biedl Syndrome and Prader-Will Syndrome. In some cases a person's genetic code and behavior may both be needed for a person to be overweight. In other cases, multiple genes may increase one's susceptibility for being overweight or obesity and require outside factors such as abundant food supply and/or little physical activity."[1]

However, factors besides genes usually determine whether or not people become overweight or obese. This next article discusses some of those other factors.

> Scientists have been working hard in an effort to identify genes that have the potential to make us fat. And it does seem there may be a genetic link to overweight and obesity—but only in a small number of people.
>
> As a result, most experts agree that while genes may have a part to play, they still don't explain the recent rapid increase in overweight that's been seen in the Western world. They believe that while we might

inherit 'fat' genes from our parents, we also inherit their bad habits such as a poor diet and lack of exercise—and it's these lifestyle factors that have a more important part to play in weight gain. This is good news for you as it means with a few lifestyle changes you should be able to shift those pounds . . .

[If] everyone in your family would benefit from losing weight, rather than going it alone, why not try and get everyone involved? While you might meet resistance from a few family members at first, once they see everyone else beginning to look slimmer, fitter, and healthier, I'm sure they be desperate to join in![2]

One of the big problems in trying to determine if genetic background or something else is influencing obesity rates is that economic status also has a strong influence. "In their review of 144 socioeconomic status/studies, it was found that the lower income levels resulted in higher levels of obesity."[3] And, to make matters worse in trying to find genetic factors, even that is changing. "Obesity, a condition that for decades has been more prevalent in the poor, is skyrocketing among affluent Americans. . . . In the 1970's, fewer than 10 percent of the most affluent were obese, compared with almost a quarter of those earning less than $25,000. In 2001-2002, just a handful of percentage points separated all income groups."[4]

Interestingly, a person's educational level also seems to have the same kinds of influences as socioeconomic status when it comes to being overweight. "The rates at which excess body weight and obesity have increased differ by level of educational attainment and gender. In general, however, individuals with lower levels of education are more likely to be overweight or obese than better educated individuals."[5]

The conclusion: genetics may very well influence either how easily you become obese, what age you start to get obese, or how obese you will become, but aside from a few rare genetic disorders, other factors will influence obesity even more. To combat all of these factors you need a calorie controlled, nutritious diet and more activity.

This brings us back to the idea of entire families being overweight. In studying these families it becomes clear that the same factors (besides genes) that influence individuals to gain weight also influence families. Surprisingly, even close friends showed this tendency to influence each other's weight.

Attitudes, behaviors, and acceptance of obesity among family and friends in a person's social network also play a strong role . . .

We were able to reconstruct a large network of individuals who had been repeatedly weighed over time . . . and we could see that as one person gained weight, those around him or her gained weight. . . .

The chance of a key participant went up by 57 percent if he, or she, had a close friend who became obese. Among pairs of brothers and sisters, one becoming obese increased the chance of the other becoming obese by 40 percent. This chance was higher among same sex siblings as opposed to opposite sex siblings. Among married couples, the chance of a husband or wife becoming obese if the spouse became obese was increased by 37 percent. Social distance, the degree of separation between two people in the network had greater influence than geographical distance. A geographical neighbor becoming obese did not increase a key participants chance of becoming obese.[6]

LOSING WEIGHT AS A FAMILY

The things necessary to get a family involved in losing weight are basically the same things needed to get an individual involved in losing weight. The main differences are that now the process involves an entire group, and that there are a few different techniques needed to get kids interested, involved, and successful in losing weight.

The ideal life portrayed on old TV shows like *Father Knows Best*, is even further from the truth now than it was back then. In that ideal life, breakfast, lunch, and dinner were all shared by the family. If that were really so, involving parents and kids in a healthy eating plan would be much easier than it is.

While adults or teens in a family may need to become involved in a weight loss program, childhood obesity in particular is becoming a grave problem. Just one concern is that overweight children are much more likely to become obese adults. Personally, I am one proof of that.

There are many helpful suggestions online for getting children involved in weight loss and healthy living.

Let's start with the kids in the family. The following section is rather long, but I include it because of the good, and fairly complete, information therein. I feel it was from the best resources I could find.

WEIGHT LOSS FOR KIDS

Getting an entire family to begin eating properly is no easy task, especially if obese children are involved. In fact, it takes far more time, attention, and effort than for just one or two members of the family. I will discuss this in greater depth later, but one of the very best motivators, before you attempt to enroll others, is to make some real headway yourself.

There are two prime reasons behind this. First, you are demonstrating that the plan actually works. Second, you will have a lot more information and expertise when it comes time to help someone else.

If you doubt how difficult it is for a family to even begin this kind of program, consider the following: "Pediatricians feel as if their efforts are futile. . . . Despite their best efforts to provide families with good advice, doctors find families lack the motivation or are so overwhelmed with the stresses of daily life that they don't attempt to attack weight problems by eating healthier and exercising more."[7] This once more brings up the subject of going to a doctor. As was advised earlier, before going on a diet consult your family doctor, especially if someone in your family is obese or has health concerns.

The following article discusses four steps for making your family more fit.

1. Create a Family Plan: The first step to becoming a fit family centers around coming together as a family. It's incredibly important to have one central health message. If one child is overweight, it's crucial that you don't isolate that individual child. Instead, make this a project that benefit's the entire family.

Sit down together and discuss everyone's favorite foods and activities. Then come up with a family plan that incorporates everyone's ideas. If one kid likes pizzas, plan a whole-wheat pizza night with all their favorite veggie toppings. If another kid likes bike rides, organize a Saturday adventure with the entire family. . .

2. Make health education a daily game: Kids are unlikely to be interested in weight-loss specifically, however, once they're engaged in planning meals or fun family activities, educating them about nutrition and fitness becomes easy. There are several low-cost products that will make education into a game, including these three:

The Funtastic Food Tracker ($19.99) allows children to record what they eat each day by placing magnetized disks on corresponding color-coded columns that represent the five major food groups. At the end of each day, the child's eating pattern can be seen at a glance, helping parents and child to make better choices.

Balance Bands ($14.95) are a visual tool to remind kids to eat their five to nine servings of fruits and vegetables every day. Each kit comes with five balance bands. To start, just put all the bracelets on your right wrist in the morning. Every time you eat a serving of fruits or veggies, you move one of the bands to your left wrist. The goal is to have all the bands on your left wrist by morning.

Neat Solutions "Weekly Exercise Chart ($5.99) is designed to motivate kids to set exercise goals and develop a sense of accomplishment. The charts break down exercise into daily boxes and include 100 sparkle-star stickers for rewarding progress.

Try setting nutrition and exercise goals for a little family-friendly competition. Then let the family member who wins pick the next meal or activity.

3. Engage kids in the kitchen: Studies show that eating a family dinner is associated with healthful dietary intake patterns, including more fruits and vegetables, less fried food and soda, less saturated and trans fat, lower glycemic load, more fiver and micronutrients from food and no material differences in red meat or snack food. Also note: Kids are more likely to eat healthy foods when they're involved in the kitchen.

The first step is to demystify the kitchen. Williams-Sonoma, for example, now makes kid-specific items such as a Kids' Chef Jacket ($42.00), Dot Vintage-Print Kids' Apron ($34.00), Dinosaur Vintage-Print Kids' apron ($34.00), Kids' Tools & Tongs Set (36.95), Kids Kitchen Tools ($39.00), and Kids' Times ($10.00). Check your local bookstore for one of the many children's cookbooks now available. Also, family cooking schools are becoming increasingly popular around the country.

Some simple ways to start include: Involving your kids in making grocery lists and shopping; having them prepare handmade menus; holding "theme" nights (for example, a Japanese night with pillows/table on the floor and dining on healthy Asian food); focusing on kid-friendly presentation such as dipping stations, taco building and carved veggies; and conducting taste tests.

4. Get your family moving: Got a family of couch potatoes? Get them moving! Physical activity can boost self-esteem and family bonding. Kids, especially those struggling with weight, like to feel like they're accepted as part of a team. Try having colored jerseys available to build team spirit. A simple relay race or impromptu game of flag football with a neighboring family can help build collegiality. Jerseys are available at most sporting goods stores.

Also try a high-tech hook. The Discovery Store sells a Discover Virtual Distance Football ($19.95) that includes a sensor that accurately determines distance the ball is thrown as well as a Discover Spy Laser Chase ($19.95) that encourages kids to play tag with a high-tech twist. Infrared "Lasers" strap to your wrist and fire quickly and accurately even when you're running. Special "Five Lives" mode lets you take five hits before you're out.

Of course, if your kids really are glued to the TV, there are some good options there, too. The Nintendo Wii "Sports" and "Boogie" ($395.96) video game encourages kids to get moving while playing one of five sports games. Disney's "High School Musical" Dance Mat ($29.99) video gets players dancing, and Fisher-Price's "Smart Cycle" ($99.99) is a great bike/video game that gets little kids moving. Both are part of Toys R Us's new "Get Up! Get Active!" campaign. Bottom line, becoming a fit family doesn't have to be painful. All it takes is some creativity and a desire to come together.[8]

In addition to these suggestions, you could try a family contest using pedometers. It could involve one pedometer that family members trade off using or one for each member of the family. There could be a reward, such as the ones mentioned in the article, for the family member who most improves the percentage of his daily record from the week before.

Remember that "if you preach to your kids about portion control, chances are they'll tune out faster than you can say Big Gulp. A better way to go is to get them involved in figuring out how much is a reasonable amount to eat."[9]

This next article gives some useful tips on how to help kids control snacking.

To avoid weight gain, keep portions small. Plan ahead and buy healthy snacks at the supermarket—you will save money and make better choices. Provide kids snack choices and make the choices you offer reasonably nutritious. Pre-portion your child's snacks into small plastic bags to grab on the go or put snack-sized servings on a plate.

For older children, designate an area in your refrigerator or cupboard for healthy snacks that you have selected and your kids like—let them help themselves without having to ask permission. Combine snacks from at least two food groups, like a protein and a carbohydrate, to pack more nutrients into your child's diets—it will be more filling and will tide them over till their next meal.

Next time you or your kids need to re-fuel, try any of the following quick, healthy snacks: string cheese and fruit (canned or fresh); nonfat cottage cheese or yogurt with fruit; smoothies with milk or yogurt and sliced bananas or strawberries; whole-wheat crackers with cheese or peanut butter; yogurt with fresh fruit or granola; low-fat chocolate milk; scoop of ice cream or frozen yogurt with fresh berries; raw vegetable sticks with low-fat yogurt dip, cottage cheese or hummus; apples and cheese—pears and other fresh fruits work too; baby carrots; fruit salad; applesauce cups (unsweetened); frozen fruit bars; dried fruit such as raisins or plums and nuts; cereal—dry or with milk; baked potato chips or tortilla chips with salsa; pretzels (lightly salted or unsalted) and a glass of milk; bagels with tomato sauce and melted cheese; flavored rice cakes (like caramel or apple cinnamon) with peanut butter; popcorn—air popped or low-fat microwave; whole-grain crackers or English muffin with peanut butter; vanilla wafers, gingersnaps, graham crackers, animal crackers or fig bars and a glass of milk.[10]

Then, there is the matter of getting kids to eat fruits and vegetables. If they are already used to these as part of their daily meals and snacks, this should not be a problem. If not, brainstorm some creative ways to get kids interested in healthy foods.

As you get ready to begin, you can determine your children's Body Mass Index by going online and typing in BMI Calculator at Keep Kids Healthy.

WEIGHT LOSS FOR TEENS

When it comes to motivating teens there are no rules. I learned this as a designer of programs for non-typical teens—teens who are about to get kicked out of school—from 1969 to 1980 and as a substitute teacher for the last few years. The most important thing to remember is that no two teens are alike; what works for one will turn another off. Even worse, stubbornness in not taking challenges that others want them to take is just one method of resistance.

However, the great news is that once teens really get into something, their energy and dedication can only be described as marvelous. This knowledge is behind every technique to interest them that I know. Almost without exception, no matter how they act or what they say, teens are insecure both about how they view themselves and what others think about them.

Anything that helps them to begin to understand who they really are, instead of who they think they are, is always the first and best step. Once they're on board, stand back, here they come! Don't just try to get them to do something. Enroll them to do all they can to accomplish it!

Are overweight teens just excessively lazy? Do they give up too quickly compared to teens who do not have weight problems? The answer to both of these questions is a resounding "No!"

Sometimes teens trying to lose weight blame themselves for having to struggle to achieve major changes in their eating and exercising habits. They say to themselves: "I am so lazy!" "I am a slob!" "I am so weak!"

However, lifestyle changes usually do involve lots of struggling. It is not laziness that makes it hard to change. The challenging nature of goals that require major changes in one's lifestyle clearly make it difficult for almost everyone. However, these difficult goals can be reached if you learn to tolerate the struggle and refuse to give up. Many people can effectively and permanently change their eating and exercising patterns. Most teenager need some help to do this, but they can get there.[11]

Another article discusses these ideas in more detail.

If your overweight teenager is ready to put some effort into getting healthier, he or she will need your help. Although gaining more independence is important to a teenager, your support is needed in this effort. You can help by creating a reasonable plan. But remember, your teen needs to buy into it and have a desire to stick with it to be successful.

Some teens do best with 1 or 2 simple goals, while others will want to move faster and make sweeping health changes. Any movement in the right direction should be encouraged. Having a partner in the plan (such as a friend) can also help. Part of being successful is to have support for when the going gets tough. . .

Tell your teen the truth. Losing weight and getting in better shape takes effort. Have open-ended conversations about the habits that lead to gaining too much weight such as not getting enough exercise, skipping meals, drinking too many soft drinks, or eating a lot of fast food. Tell your teen about how weight and body shape run in families. . . .

People eat for many reasons such as time of day, boredom, or feeling frustrated, nervous or depressed. The best reason to eat is hunger. Ask your teen (what is going on with them and why they do it) when they eat, overeat, or crave certain foods. If your teen is eating when not hungry, encourage your teen to do something else to get food off of the mind such as exercising, reading or working on a project.

Help your teen practice eating until comfortable, not stuffed. If your teen eats until comfortable, he should be hungry every 2 - 3 hours. Snacking is not a bad habit, as long as snacks are healthy . . .[12]

Many teens today have a hectic lifestyle.

Both the food and the enjoyment kids get out of preparing and eating meals can help enhance the appeal of healthful eating. Here are some guidelines to help get your teen on track: Skipping breakfast is a big mistake, but teens often do it. "I don't have time," "I'm not hungry," "I'd rather sleep," or "I hate breakfast food" are just a few of the excuses teen use to avoid eating in the morning. Breakfast is essential for a healthful diet.

These tips may help teens to work this important meal into their busy schedules: Offer granola bars, bananas, and other breakfast foods that can be eaten on the bus or in the car. Keep it simple. Include a protein, complex carbohydrate, and a fruit; cereal with milk and fruit or a bagel with peanut butter and an apple to eat on the way to school. Make your own "fast food." Bake fruit and oatmeal bars with your teen on the weekend, so they'll be ready to grab during the week. Get creative. Pretty much any food can be a breakfast food: leftovers from last night's dinner, a sandwich, cottage cheese and fruit, or whatever your kid will eat.

Encourage teens to try new foods. Today, more than ever, we have an enormous array of healthful—and even exotic—foods from which to choose. . .

Bring them grocery shopping and have them pick some new foods for your family to try. Encourage the whole family to try new fruit or vegetables each week, such as mango, and spaghetti squash. Try ethnic cuisines—Thai, Mexican, Moroccan, Spanish, Japanese, etc.

Mix favorite foods with not-so-favorite foods. For example, most kids like cereal, smoothies, pasta, and sandwiches; here are some ideas for boosting the nutrition in these foods: Stock your pantry with a variety of cereals—some high fiber choices and some lower-fiber, high-sugar cereals that teens tend to favor. Suggest that your teen combine a high-fiber cereal with their usual cereal for their morning bowl. They'll still taste the sweetness and get some extra nutrients. Encourage kids to add sliced fresh fruit (blueberries, bananas or strawberries) or dried fruit (raisins, dried cranberries, dried dates) to a bowl of cereal.

Smoothies are popular among teens. Make these drinks with skim milk, or juice, frozen yogurt or light ice cream, and fruit. Stir fry fresh or frozen vegetables in olive oil and toss them with pasta and tomato sauce.

Add sesame seeds, fruit, raisins, scallions, or other nontraditional salad ingredients to liven up a green salad. Stuff sandwiches with cucumber and tomato slices, lettuce or spinach leaves, and sprouts, and use smaller amounts of meat and cheese.

Tailor meal times to energy needs. Because of their busy lifestyles, teens' diets need to be tailored to their schedules. For kids with sports or jobs after school, provide them with a hearty snack, such as a peanut butter sandwich and an apple to eat before heading off to practice or work. If extracurricular activities interfere with dinner time, have leftovers ready when your teen gets home. Make healthful entrees on the weekend and freeze them in individual containers that can be thawed and heated for quick dinners during the week. Keep the kitchen, school locker, and backpack well stocked with healthful snacks . . .[13]

One final article gives the following advice.

[Discuss with] your teen why eating too much junk food is unhealthy. It can make them gain weight, effect his energy and mood levels and can negatively impact his academic performance. Discuss reasons why choosing healthy food over junk food makes sense. Eating healthy snacks counteracts the negative effects of eating junk. Explain that healthy doesn't have to equal bland or bad-tasting. There are plenty of nutritious and delicious alternatives.

Shop with your teen. Encourage her to read labels and discuss the nutritional content of her favorite foods. Explore healthy alternatives that she enjoys or is at least willing to try.

Make healthy snacks. . . . Model healthy snack habits by limiting your own intake of junk food. If your teen sees you eating healthy snacks, he will be more apt to follow your lead. Provide encouragement to your teen as she tries to break the junk food habit. It will be difficult at times, but with your support she will succeed.[14]

Many of the same tips for involving kids apply to teens and vice versa. For both children and teens the key is to enroll them in changing things that will improve their lives. Telling them won't do, advising them won't do, coaxing them won't do, threatening them won't do and arguing with them certainly won't do.

There are a number of steps in enrolling people to make changes. One is to ask questions about what they want, what makes them happy, and what discourages them. Make it obvious that the discussion is about them, not what you want them to do. If they seem to become at least partially enrolled, then it might be time to ask what they want to do or accomplish and how you can support them. Then, and only then, it might be appropriate to begin using some of the tips mentioned in the articles above.

It might not be a bad idea, in the case of teens, to let them read this part of the book, which is about them—if they want to. Then if they really get on board, have them read the whole book.

LOSING WEIGHT AS A FAMILY

The title of one diet book is *Lean Mom, Fit Family.*[15] The truth in this statement is that one thinner person in the family can motivate everyone else. I know that in my life, for years I never wanted to hear about the latest diet craze, let alone try it. I was, however, interested when someone I knew lost large amounts of fat. When others in the family began to have good success on the RMR diet, I was intrigued enough to try it myself.

Unless the other adults in your family are already highly motivated, the best way to interest them might well be to get rid of enough fat to begin to change your appearance. Nearly all overweight people want to change how they look, and seeing someone else do it can inspire them.

It was not until I actually tried it myself that I discovered how easy, with respect to not being hungry throughout the day, all this could be. I hate to keep throwing in words like landmark, but properly understood, that is the only way to describe the wonderful results.

In short, if you want to get someone else involved in the RMR diet, first let them see how much fat you are burning, and then allow them to begin questioning you about it. If that doesn't work, here are some other tools that might help.

When your family members see you enjoying a whole new variety of snacks, this by itself can inspire interest. Soon, almost certainly, they will be partaking of these delicacies themselves without even considering the word "diet." I know I did. Letting them share your snacks can be fun for two reasons. First, because you enjoy seeing them doing what you do, and second, because you anticipate what is coming next.

One thing is for certain. They will notice you weighing things and recording your calories. If they ask about this, "I'm on a new type of diet," will suffice. Their willingness to try it may or may not occur at this time. No matter what transpires, sooner or later, those with a weight problem will begin questioning you—and they will probably get on the program themselves.

It may not happen until after you've burned enough fat that it becomes noticeable, and that will take time. But what's the rush, right? You've got the rest of your life.

As you try to involve others in your RMR plans, remember that most people with a weight problem are sensitive about it. I was. Bobbie never had to mention that I was fat and needed to go on a diet. I'd already known that for decades. She just showed me the way.

I am spending more time on this concept than some might like, but I do it for a good reason. Once you do get others involved, and they started producing results in their lives, it will be one more great and enjoyable thing about the RMR diet for you. I have always been extremely happy when I see the good that the RMR diet has done for others.

Whether the other members of your family have a weight problem or not, cooking special meals for them can be fun for you. But more important, if you cook the meal in a low-fat, nutritious way, as outlined in this book, you help them on their way to a healthier lifestyle. This applies whether it is for your spouse, your children, or friends you invited in.

It doesn't matter whom you invite for a special occasion—enjoyment is the order of the day. Special meals like this can help you increase the bonds between you and the ones you love. This is not only important, it is vital. You can create special occasions for a great meal in addition to your existing traditions. An anniversary is just one example. Remembering to celebrate special occasions with appropriate, healthy meals will make your RMR plan more successful and enjoyable.

When I was younger, making a million dollars and having a Rolls Royce seemed important. Now, good health and enjoying time with my family top the list. Having a Rolls Royce is nothing in comparison to having a healthy, happy family. Properly used, the RMR diet can get you both more in touch with your family and create more enjoyment for all of you.

Eating at Different Times of the Year

Often our bodies will prompt us to eat lightly in the summer, or gorge on heavy foods in the winter without our ever being aware of it.

A vital way to control what and how much you eat is to question the desires you have to eat a particular item or dish. If what you want is appropriate to the season, fine. But if you find yourself just dying for mashed potatoes in the middle of the summer, you should try to identify what is behind that urge, just in case the cause of your craving is something sinister like depression.

Being aware of season-appropriate desires means we need not look so closely at the motivation behind such desires. Identifying the cause of your cravings will help you to stay on the path you've chosen for yourself.

One of the advantages to listening to your body's cravings is that you will eat a larger variety of foods as the seasons change. Not only is this more nutritious than eating the same thing all the time, but it also tends to satisfy something inside you.

Fall

Since ancient times, our bodies have instinctively begun to bulk up in fall in preparation for the coming cold. Why fall? That's when the greatest harvest of bulk-up foods occurred.

This may mean that even if you've been doing fine on the RMR diet, when fall begins you might suddenly begin to feel that you're just not getting enough to eat. If this happens you have two main choices. The first is to recognize this phenomenon and continue eating as you have for a few days, gradually reducing your intake back down to a normal level. Another option is to choose seasonal foods that are low in calories, like squash.

Winter

Winter has traditionally been a time to continue to bulk up on heavier foods in preparation for the coming cold. Another problem is that there are fewer outdoor activities. Therefore, we should give attention to what will help us continue to burn fat.

In ancient times our bodies kept us alive in the cold by turning food into heat. The body really does have its own thermostat. As temperatures go down, fuel consumption goes up.

These days, most of us do not have to worry about freezing to death in the winter, except in some rare emergency. Though we don't have to worry about cold, the nutritional value of traditional winter foods still applies. It might well be wise to indulge yourself in some of these foods you crave in winter, such as hearty soups, beans, and other warming foods. I've found that a cup full of them, along with lighter fare such as cooked veggies to fill up on, works very well.

With your body craving these hearty foods, it's no surprise that this is the time of year most people go off their diets. Understanding and accepting what each time of the year brings in terms of cravings can help you to cope with those seasonal changes. If you suddenly find yourself eating more than the RMR limit in the winter, remembering how the seasons affect your diet could well make the difference between staying on your plan, or ending up right back where you started.

Spring

In the spring you may suddenly find you have the desire for a great salad. Why? Again because of history. Spring is the time of year most salad foods first become available. In the old days when these weren't available all year round, our bodies craved them in the spring to stave off diseases like scurvy and beri beri.

Summer

Light food is the hallmark of summer eating. This includes fruits. Light foods are the norm, especially on the hottest days. Studies have shown more people go on diets in the summer than at any other time of the year.

The diet food and exercise equipment industries know this. Frequently you will see women in scanty bathing suits proclaiming they have "shaped up," for summer. Of course they're doing it by buying the product the commercial is touting.

The Holiday Season

Can you guess which season is the most difficult for any dieter? Yes, it's the holiday season. This is one of the most dangerous times of the year in terms of remaining on our diets.

It doesn't matter whether we're talking about Thanksgiving, Christmas, or New Year's, this time of year always seems to include large family gatherings and enough food on the table to feed the underprivileged in Kenya for a month.

In times past I made it through Thanksgiving pretty well, but Christmas was just too much for me. On the RMR diet, I had to use every trick in the book during my first holiday season. My daily calorie record for such days, before I learned to handle them, used to include no calorie listings, but did contain the phrase, "blew it." On some days, I still don't have the foggiest idea how many calories a particular dish contains—and I don't care.

However I have noticed that just knowing what I do about the principles of the RMR diet means that blowing it now only involves eating less than half the calories I used to consume when I would blow it before. And, since I slowed my eating rate, I've found that even during the holidays I don't blow it as often and I can calculate, or closely estimate, what I ate.

Activities for Every Season

Unless you live in the Gobi desert, you will probably have to adjust your activity habits at different times of the year. Few of us go skiing in August, at least in the Northern Hemisphere. The nice thing about the RMR diet is that what you do matters less than the fact that you're doing something.

The reason you need to pay attention to the time of year is to make sure you don't let these natural changes of seasons stop you from being active. Naturally, if you try the "no more commercials" routine, that could be carried out all year long. However, even then, you might want to do different activities in the summer than you did in the winter. It really doesn't matter what you do as long as you do something active at every time of the year.

So what's the lesson? Listen to your body. It has learned how to vary your diet throughout the different times of the year to get optimum nutrition, and prepare you for the specific activities each season brings.

Notes

1. "Obesity and Genetics—How do genes affect obesity?" http://www.weight-awareness.com/topics/doc.xml?doc_id=1187&_topic_id=111.
2. Juliette Kellow, B.Sc., R.D., "Overweight and Genetics" http://www.weightlossresources.co.uk/body_weight/overweight/genetics.htm.
3. Tommer Yoked, "Fat and Getting Fatter" www.tcnj.edu/~business/economics/documents/T_Yoked.thesis.pdf.
4. Nanci Hellmich, "Obesity Surges Among Affluent," *USAToday.com,* http://www.usatoday.com/news/health/2005-05-02-obesity-affluent_x.htm.
5. Joanne Appleton-Arnaud, Ph.D, "Parental Education Key to Health for Parents and Children," http://www.pubmedcentral.nih.gov/articlerender.fcgi?artid=2396984.

6. "Obesity Spreads Among Friends and Family," http://www.mededicalnewstoday.com/articles/77889.php.

7. "Pediatricians Say Advice to Obese Kids and Families Falls On Deaf Ears," http://www.eurekalert.org/pub_releases/2007-07/slu-psa071607.php.

8. Joy Bauer, MS, RD, CDN, "4 Simple Steps to Make Your Family a Fit Family," msnbc.com, http://today.msnbc.msn.com/id/21412486/.

9. "Keeping Portions Under Control," http://kidshealth.org/parent/food/weight/portions.html#.

10. "Smart Snacking Tips for Children," http://www.mealsmatter.org/CookingForFamily/Planning/article.aspx?articleId=43.

11. "Is My Teen Just Lazy?" http://www.4teenweightloss.com/teen-motivation.html.

12. "Helping Your Overweight Teen," www.sandburgptsa.org/committees/overweight.pdf.

13. "Healthful Eating for Teens on the Run," http://www.upmc.com/HealthAtoZ/Pages/HealthLibrary.aspx?chunkiid=14396.

14. "How To Get Your Teen Off Junk Food," http://www.ehow.com/how_2177416_teen-off-junk-food.html.

15. This book is by Michael Sena, Kirsten Straughan and Thomas P. Sattler. It contains "A 6-week plan for a slimmer you and a healthier family." I can neither recommend, nor condemn it because I have not read it. Although I do wonder about any plan that can be handled in six weeks, unless that is just a start for a lifelong change, which, I imagine, is their philosophy.

13

Pitfalls and Slippery Slopes

Slippery slopes are not usually dangerous. All of us have encountered slippery slopes of one kind or another, whether it's in a city on an icy driveway or out in the country on a wet grassy knoll. Usually, we discover them with our feet slipping out from under us and we know a fall is on the way. We didn't know it was coming, or we would have been far more careful.

Often that fall only hurts a little and most of the damage is done to our pride. Sometimes, especially as we get older, it can result in serious injury to the back or hip. Rarely are such falls fatal, but they can be.

Pitfalls are another matter. Most of them can be very dangerous. If you look up *pitfall* in *Roget's Thesaurus* you will find the related words: *drawback, snare, snag, danger, downside, consequence, difficulty,* and *hazard.*

In the past when I began diets, things would go reasonably well at first. No matter how difficult or uncomfortable it was, my determination and willpower would triumph.

But then, either quickly or after a longer time, something would happen and that would be the end of that. Whether it happened slowly, like sliding down a grassy hillside or suddenly like plunging into a pitfall, the result was always the same: bye-bye to my hopes, dreams, and the healthy benefits the diet could have provided.

Many little problems that arise while dieting have already been covered in this book. But nowhere have they been listed all together, so that you can read the list and remember them. Now is the time for that.

The images of slippery slopes and pitfalls help you visualize what happens to you when you find one. In the physical world, if that driveway is icy, you know to use extreme caution. If that grassy hillside is wet, you plant one foot firmly before taking the next step. On our diets, recognizing these dangers and taking appropriate steps to prevent a fall is equally important.

The term "slippery slope" will be reserved for littler problems that are dangerous only if you don't recognize them and regain your balance before you fall. A pitfall will be used for dangers that can kill your diet if you don't stay vigilant and recognize that you're in danger before you fall into one.

Not every problem covered in the book will be repeated here. The purpose of this section is to list the ones that are potentially the most dangerous and, more important, to put them all in one place so they can be recognized and remembered.

SLIPPERY SLOPES

This next section will list some of the slippery slopes you may encounter on the RMR diet. Recognizing these dangers can help you to avoid them or to rectify the situation when you do encounter them.

The "I've been doing good" Slippery Slope

When a special occasion comes up you might tell yourself "I've been doing good, so it won't hurt to blow it today." And it doesn't—unless those special days start coming closer and closer together.

Something special might include a dish you love, going out to eat, or cooking something good for a get-together with other members of the family.

One of the ways I learned to handle this slippery slope was to tell myself, "Yeah, I've been doing good—and I'm going to keep on doing good."

The "I Forgot" Slippery Slope

It's time for a snack and I eat it, but I'm not paying attention since I have other things on my mind. Too busy to record it, I tell myself, "I'll do it later." But I don't. Then, I completely forget I've eaten it. By the time my calorie count is totaled for the day and I've matched my RMR, in truth, I've overeaten. Using "I forgot" as an excuse does not change what happened. You're still over your caloric limit for the day.

But, possibly as bad, I haven't enjoyed what I've eaten in such cases.

Not savoring what you eat is just another form of unconscious eating. Remember, a meal (or snack) savored is one that satisfies. If you notice yourself rushing a snack to the point that you don't even record it, slow down! Take a deep breath and exhale slowly. Then savor the snack and take the time to record it.

Recording everything as soon as it's eaten can be one problem in following the RMR diet. Often, it's a pain in the neck, you are rushed to clean up after a meal, or something comes up. Your mind will look for an easier way—but there isn't one!

Accepting that this is one lifestyle change you will simply have to learn to live with will actually help you to continue doing it. Not recording now and then is not a big problem. But if it becomes a habit, use the three-week habit replacement program to change your ways.

The Family Gatherings Slippery Slope

There are three reasons family gatherings or any group setting involving food can be a problem.

1. You are so busy chatting that you're not really concentrating on your plan.
2. There are so many good things available. In my family most of them are pies, cakes, and different flavors of ice cream.
3. You don't want others to notice how small your portions are, or that you've slowed your rate of eating.

If you've got to blow it at a family gathering, do your very best to limit the damage you do. For example, satisfy yourself with one of the sweets—not all of them.

The Slippery Slope of Going Out to Eat

Going out to eat too often or eating too much when you do go out are two of the real dangers on an eating plan. Handling this slippery slope should be pretty high on your habit replacement list. Try working on it as soon as you've replaced enough of your other troublesome habits to be able to handle it without much trouble.

The Slippery Slope of Cheating

Cheating on your diet doesn't have to be a big problem. Just forgive yourself and get back on your diet. Whatever you do, though, don't let cheating become a habit. But if you do, replace that habit with the three-week habit replacement program.

The "Let's have another" Slippery Slope

More than one snack at a time probably isn't a snack. It may be getting close to a meal. Too many snacks can cause problems when meal time comes. You might have to cut down your calorie intake at your next meal so that you don't exceed your RMR limit.

Waiting the appropriate time after a snack so that your feeling of satisfaction can kick in, is something that is very helpful. On rare occasions, when the appropriate time for your feeling of hunger to be gone has passed, but your hunger hasn't, another, smaller, snack may be appropriate. Of course, if you make the second snack something like carrots, quantity will not be such a big deal, and you won't have to cut down your meal either.[1]

The Slippery Slope of Between-Meal Appetites

This slippery slope ties directly into the one listed above it, but there is a slight difference. What we're discussing now is if you begin feeling appetite often between meals. There is a real and important difference between genuine hunger and mere appetite.

If you notice you are feeling this appetite between meals at certain times, plan a little snack just before the time it usually sets in. If you still experience them, try increasing how much you eat at the meals before they occur. Remember eating more does not necessarily mean eating more calories. More veggies or fruit may take care of it.

The Slippery Slope of Not Eating Enough

Not eating enough is itself a slippery slope that can hurt you. If, now and then, we do not meet our caloric limit and no strong appetites kick in, no problem. But frequently not eating enough shifts this problem rapidly from a slope to a pitfall. It is dangerous for many reasons. One danger is entering starvation mode, and another is poor nutrition, both of which are harmful to your health.

The Slippery Slope of Unconscious Eating

Eating unconsciously doesn't mean you're losing your memory or can't focus your thoughts. Most of us have actually eaten unconsciously for years. It was there, we grabbed it off the counter and—pop—into our mouths it went without us even realizing we had done it.

This is a problem that often occurs early in the program. Obviously, if it is allowed to go unchecked, it will sabotage all you want and need from your RMR experience. And you may not even know why!

Such a lifelong habit requires a lot of concentration when you first take it on for replacement. If you have a problem remembering to control it, try following the tip already mentioned about putting something easily noticeable out of place to remind you. For example, in the cupboard, you could place a large empty can on its side at eye level. Then when you open the cupboard—that darn can will be staring you right in the eye. In the fridge, a large bottle filled with outlandishly colored water could be placed at eye level where it won't be missed. Let's say you've got some trail mix in a bowl on the counter. Until you can resist taking it unconsciously, cover it with a sheet of folded newspaper.

The "No snacks available" Slippery Slope

In snacking, speed can sometimes be important. Obviously, the quicker you take care of an appetite urging, the less chance it will have to do you damage. In fact, many times I now even find a little pleasure in experiencing appetite and getting a snack to handle it.

The longer it takes you to get something to snack on, the longer your appetites will gnaw at you. The only answer is to have a number of snacks available at all times. Having many different types of snacks on hand will also help you to maintain your nutritional needs.

An additional tip is to have both low-calorie and moderate-calorie snacks available. If your meals that day have been a little high in calories, you can use the low-calorie snacks. Conversely, if your meals have been a little low in calories, you can grab one of your moderate-calorie snacks to handle the appetite.

For me, this can be as simple as deciding whether I take the lower-calorie feta cheese or the higher calorie cheddar cheese. At other times, when I've had a few more calories, it might just be green olives, a pickle, or some baby carrots.

The Slippery Slope of Hypoglycemia

This is a new one we haven't discussed before. Most people think hypoglycemia is only a problem for diabetics. However, it actually affects almost everyone at times—especially people on diets. Hypoglycemia occurs when your blood sugar or the glucose levels in your blood fall below what you need to nourish your cells. When this happens, one way your body reacts is to produce an excess of insulin to help maintain your system.

In healthy people this drop in blood sugar levels can have numerous causes. One is insufficient food intake. Another is going too long between meals or snacks. And still another is increased physical activity to the point that the body can't burn fat quickly enough to keep up with blood sugar needs.

One common example of how this can happen waking up in the morning and getting busy before getting your body its needed nourishment. Hypoglycemia can also set in when you go a long time between meals and snacks, or if you participate in some extra physical activity. This is one reason all health experts insist that breakfast is the most important meal of the day.

You need not trouble yourself about trying to determine whether your blood sugar is getting too low. Your body will tell you. It's more of a problem to recognize it when it happens. The key thing is noticing when all of a sudden, and for no reason you are aware of, you get "way off center."

Personally, I discover I am getting hypoglycemic symptoms in two ways. The first is that I may notice I'm getting agitated. "Agitated at what?" you might ask. Everything! The second symptom I notice is that I run out of steam and begin feeling extra tired. My body will always tell me when to slow down and let it catch up in its fat burning process.

Hypoglycemia in non-diabetics can disappear about as fast as it came on if you recognize it and take appropriate action. Actually, one sure way to get rid of it is to do nothing. If you sit and do nothing for awhile, your body will burn a little fat, deposit the glucose into your blood stream, and then you'll be ready to go again.

But the quickest cure for hypoglycemia is a snack, a little sugary sweet something, or one of the easier-to-digest carbohydrates. Then give your body a little time to react. A snack is good because even if the glucose from fat does start flowing again after a rest, further activity just makes the next outbreak come quicker. An appropriate snack can forestall that. Once your snack is being processed, you can again be active without hypoglycemia reoccurring.

This article discusses hypoglycemia in more detail.

> Hypoglycemia, also called low blood sugar, occurs when your blood glucose (blood sugar) level drops too low to provide enough energy for your body's activities. . . . Glucose, a form of sugar, is an important fuel for your body. Carbohydrates are the main dietary sources of glucose. Rice, potatoes, bread, tortillas, cereal, milk fruit, and sweets are all carbohydrate-rich foods . . .

Symptoms of hypoglycemia include: hunger; nervousness and shakiness; perspiration; dizziness or light-headedness; sleeplessness; confusion; difficulty sleeping; feeling anxious or weak. Hypoglycemia can also happen while you are sleeping. You might: cry out or have nightmares; find that your pajamas or sheets are damp from perspiration; or feel tired, irritable or confused when you wake up.[2]

The Slippery Slope of Packaged Foods

Sometimes it just isn't convenient or you don't have time to prepare everything from scratch. At such times, prepackaged foods that you can just mix together and heat up for a few minutes or throw in the microwave are a blessing.

Unfortunately, many prepackaged foods are just too darn high in calories. If you don't think these foods can be a disaster to a diet, just read the labels on a few and judge for yourself. In fact, that is the key to preventing this slippery slope. Make sure you know both the calories in, and how much you can have of, any packaged food. Especially one you've been using for years and never checked.

I still use my favorite prepackaged foods sometimes, but I'm very aware of making them just one part of my meal and eating only a small portion to keep my calories within my RMR limit.

Eating only a small portion of your favorite prepackaged food might seem like a waste of both time and taste. Not so! One of the best things about the RMR diet is that you can eat anything you really want—in moderation. Learning to satisfy yourself with a smaller amount of your favorite high-calorie foods will actually let you enjoy them more, since you won't have to feel guilty about eating them. The slippery slope occurs when you do as I have so often done in the past and eat far more of these packaged foods than you should be eating.

The Slippery Slope of Taking the Whole Package

"Lets see," I think to myself, "three Doritos are thirty-six calories. That sounds good." Then I grab the whole package and head to the couch to watch TV. You know the rest. And, obviously, we're not just talking about Doritos here. The same thing can happen with crackers, nuts, potato chips, candy, baby marshmallows, or anything else from a package that you can only take a small amount of.

Two tips can help with this slippery slope: include a measuring scoop in the package, or take out the right amount and put it in individual baggies.

If you use the second tip, all you will need do is grab a baggie—the package is gone. And if you grab for a second baggie you will know that you're adding those excess calories. The first tip will not control your intake as effectively as individual baggies, but it will help. If the item in the package needs measuring, at least put the appropriate measuring device in it, such as a tablespoon or a measuring cup, depending on what the proper portion is.

The Slippery Slope of Eating When Upset

Eating when you're upset is different from emotional eating, which is a pitfall and will be covered later. What we are discussing now is that everyone gets upset sometimes, and sometimes you might get upset several times in one day. The key to handling this slippery slope is to recognize why you are upset. Are you angry? Disappointed about something? Frustrated? Grieving about something or someone? Whatever it is, you're upset and you need to recognize that you are upset.

You cannot let the fact that you are upset cause you to overeat. Actually, this is a fairly simple process in mild cases. Split your upset feelings and your eating into two separate events. Say to yourself, "I'm upset. I will not let that cause me to overeat." If you're really distraught there are a couple of possibilities. One is not to eat until the feeling leaves. The second is to be very careful when you're measuring your portions, and to not take seconds.

The Slippery Slope of Isolation

Feeling isolated is one of those emotions that can make us unhappy and dissatisfied. This can really take away from some of the successes and joys that can occur on this plan. Being isolated during your RMR diet can, by itself, cause problems. The most important problem is the tendency to not seek help or comfort to help you deal with any part of the diet that is causing you problems. It really works to have a buddy, but even if you don't, do your best to find a friend, sibling, parent, or someone else you can call when you need to discuss something.

To handle this slippery slope, notify those around you about why you're doing what you are doing, especially when your eating practices are sure to make them notice and wonder what is going on. The first thing to announce is that you are going on a diet. This need not be a big or dramatic thing. For example, during dinner you might say something like, "I've been eating too much lately. I think I'll go on a diet."

Then, as appropriate, or if you get questioning stares, you might want to explain such things as why you are measuring things, why you're putting snacks in baggies, why you're taking smaller portions, and why you're eating more slowly. If you explain your reasoning, you may be surprised at how supportive the people around you will be.

The Slippery Slope of a Lack of Knowledge

Every effort has been made with this book to make the RMR diet a complete plan and give you all the information you might need. Some might argue there is too much information. That, however, is because we are all unique individuals, and there is no way to know in advance just what you will and will not need. Better to have too much information and let you disregard what doesn't interest you than to give many people too little information.

However, it is possible that there is something in this book that you do not understand completely. In such cases, do not let this discourage you or stop you from succeeding. Use some of the sources for information that have already been mentioned. Chief among these are books, the Internet, and a friend you can discuss things with who might be able to help you get what you need.

PITFALLS

As was mentioned, pitfalls are a snare or a trap. Once you are really into one, there may be no way out but the death of the diet. That's why extra effort in watching for them pays off. And if they start to trap you, get out quick! This may sound melodramatic, but it's not. There are many studies showing that a huge percentage of people who go on a diet fail. Don't let it happen to you! Use this list of pitfalls to recognize impending danger and take action immediately.

The Pitfall of Expecting Too Much Too Soon

You can expect this one near the start of a diet, and near the end as well. You do all you need to do to get going, and then you wait for the good results that will make all that effort worth it. And you wait some more. And finally you decide that the little bit that is happening just is not worth it.

But take heart; remember this eating plan is a lifelong thing. It is not one of those quick weight loss schemes like the high-protein low-carb diets we discussed earlier.

One of the huge benefits in losing no more than a pound (or two at the most) in a week is that many serious problems such as the starvation mode and illness related to poor nutrition do not occur with the RMR diet.

The other time when this pitfall will begin to effect you is six months to a year from when you begin. By then you may have become tired of still having to pay so much attention to what, how much, and when you eat after such a long period of time. The expecting "too much" applies here as well because the closer you get to your goal weight, the slower the weight will be coming off. Instead of a pound or two a week, you might now be down to a pound or two a month.

Discouragement will be covered shortly as its own pitfall, but at the bottom line of this pitfall is that you become discouraged. If you don't consciously quit dieting outright, then you just stop concentrating on what needs to be done. The actual quitting will occur over time. And then this will be just one more diet that failed.

The Pitfall of Serious Emotional Eating

From previous discussions and experiences you know that most people have used food to relieve certain strong emotions, and you also know some tips for how to overcome that tendency. But now we are talking about heavy emotional eating that you cannot seem to control no matter what you do.

In short, we're speaking about neuroses or psychoses. The only help for psychosis is a psychiatric expert. A neurosis might also call for that if it is a particularly strong one, but many neuroses can be helped by talking with a close friend, a diet buddy, or your family physician.

While you might not know which of the above is plaguing you, you can be reasonably certain something serious is preventing you from living the kind of life you want to. Only you can decide whether such help is needed or even possible for you.

One thing you can know, however, is that unless this pitfall is handled it will cause you problems for the rest of your life. That being true, now might be a good time to get help if you need it.

The Pitfall of Depression

Being in a state of deep depression can make the RMR diet and everything else in your life a downer. Clinical depression should be discussed with your doctor. Perhaps an anti-depression drug is in order. Given the vagaries of life, things happen to all of us that might well lead to being depressed for awhile. One of my common practices in the past to handle depression was to eat. Don't ask me why. I don't know why. All I know is that's what I did.

If, in milder cases, you suddenly feel the urge to eat, remember, it will pass. For more serious episodes, being aware of this depression pitfall can be like raising a red flag. The flag signals: Don't go off your RMR diet! Don't go off your RMR diet!

The Pitfall of Stress

To deal with this pitfall, reread the information for the previous pitfall and substitute stress for depression. They both have the same effect, and being aware of that effect is vital.

The Pitfall of Starvation Mode

This one is really a big bad bear. When the starvation mode has been going on long enough, our bodies will make it clear to us that they have had enough of it. If we're too stupid to know we're starving and starting to damage things, our bodies are not. They'll do whatever it takes to make sure they get nourished again, which can definitely result in the end of a diet.

Preventing this pitfall is so critical that if you do not remember the signs of it, and how relatively easy it is to cure, you might want to reread the information that was given about it earlier.

The Pitfall of "What's the Use?"

Emotional, depressed, and stress eating can make you ask yourself, what's the use? Sometimes you may begin to feel it's all hopeless. You know in the end it really isn't, but that doesn't help much in curing those feelings. The only solution is not to let your thoughts ruin one of the main things in your life that can give you hope and vitality—your health!

If you're a pessimist, when it comes to diets, you will have to watch out for this one even closer. Find ways to keep reminding yourself of the benefits of the RMR diet and the things that can make it a wonderful experience.

The Pitfall of "I've Already Blown It"

With this pitfall we're not talking about blowing it for an occasional meal or a day. We are speaking about having blown it for a week or a month.

This one is easy to recognize because you will know you are no longer dieting, even though you might still be doing a few things to try to control your eating. That's when recognizing this pitfall can make all the difference in the world.

Beginning the RMR diet again even after such a long time can still revolutionize your health, vitality, and life.

The Pitfall of Portion Creep

When portion creep occurs during the fat-burning part of your eating plan, your scale will show you it is happening and correcting it will be reasonably easy. If you're not measuring portions, start again. If you're estimating portions, cut down the sizes of what you're using for estimates.

This pitfall only turns into a death trap after the fat burning part of the eating plan is completed and you shift over to eating your BMR calories instead. If you allow it to go unchecked, your "diet" will have been successful, but you will end up right back where you started.

Just as your scale will let you know if portion control is a problem during the fat-burning process, it will also let you know if it is happening while you are eating your BMR calories. Once you've lost all the weight you want to, you might decide to stop weighing yourself because what the scale says is no longer so important. Wrong! For the rest of your life you should weigh yourself at least once per month.

Not only will this let you know if you're letting your portions creep up on you, but as a part of your overall health you should be on the lookout for either weight loss or weight gain once you are eating a stable diet. Many health problems are signaled by a sudden weight drop or gain.

The Pitfall of Genetics

As has previously been mentioned, the genetics excuse used to be framed as, "My whole family is overweight. We are just born that way." Scientists might agree with that statement, but they would modify it to something like, "Since most of my family is overweight, it seems we have a genetic tendency to weigh more than we should."

We have already covered some new evidence showing that there can be a genetic component in weight gain and what to do about it. If such genetic tendencies are found in your family, all the more care needs to be taken to prevent obesity and its attendant health problems. In other words, not only is such a genetic link not an excuse, it is a warning sign and must be used to correct being overweight.

The Pitfall of Other Excuses

Occasionally some new excuse will creep out from your subconscious and make itself felt. Whether it is one of the pitfalls already mentioned or one unique to you, there is no reason to let a pitfall, or anything else, stop you from your dreams.

NOTES

1. In spite of what you just read about recording everything you eat, if I have a few baby carrots, a pickle, a couple of sticks of celery, or any other ultra-low-calorie snack, I don't bother to record it. When I get up around twenty-five calories, like for five green olives, however, that goes on my records.
2. "Hypoglycemia" http://diabetes.niddk.nih.gov/dm/pubs/hypoglycemia/.

Conclusion

Since you've stuck with it this far, you have demonstrated you have the desire and will to do all that needs to be done. Good for you!

In many ways you will find it is easier to actually do the RMR diet than read about it. If you've already done some of the hard part, you will do the rest. When talking about teens, I mentioned that once they were enrolled, get out of their way. I know you are enrolled because you got this far. So, the same goes for you. I am about to get out of your way!

I've learned many important lessons in life. One is that most people are far smarter, far more capable, and far more dedicated than they realize. If you have any doubts in this area, just trust me. Get started and soon you'll have a whole new opinion of what you can and cannot do.

I can offer you no greater encouragement than to point out that if, after a lifetime of trying and failing, an old geezer like me can do it, anybody can do it. I have learned that the life changes the RMR diet brings about far outweigh any effort needed to do it. Can you see that the results of health and enjoyment in your life will be experienced for a long, long, long time? That alone should be reason enough for you to succeed.

I hope you are now aware of something that will change and improve your life from this point on. Starting today, you'll achieve your weight loss dreams, increase your vitality, improve your health, and contribute to your life. It is founded on personal experience, experiences of others, science, and the latest research. You can have faith in it.

To help you get started, I want to review the basics. First, you'll need to calculate your RMR. As your weight goes down, you will be burning less energy and will need to recalculate your RMR. You can anticipate that once you are eating within your RMR limit, every single thing you do will burn fat, even if it is only getting out of one chair and sitting in another.

Remember that this is a plan you will tailor to fit you as a unique individual. The more familiar you are with this book, the better you can make the RMR diet fit your needs, and the more certain you'll be of success. Also remember that this is a gradual, painless plan that you can ease into.

You'll need to get measuring spoons and cups, a small scale for measuring such things as meat and cheese, and a scale to weigh yourself on. You will need a good calorie counting book, a journal for recording your weight, thoughts, plans, and questions. You will need forms for logging in your daily portions and calories, unless you are going to record them in your journal or track them electronically.

You will need to begin planning how you will stay within your RMR limit and make sure you are coming close to following the Food Guide Pyramid. If you have any problems with any of this you can review the appropriate sections in this book.

You will need to start slow and easy, implementing only a couple of parts of the plan at a time. Don't add more until you're comfortable with the ones you've already begun.

While you're doing this you can begin logging your accomplishments into your journal along with what you're having trouble with and how you are feeling from day to day. Then, you can start a section on planning. Review some of the things you might consider planning. As you plan, remember the Goal Approach Quotient, which can be used to supply you with extra motivation.

You also need to be aware of certain problems that may arise such as the starvation mode, plateaus, and others. If you do have problems, both the problem and what you plan to do about it should also go in your journal.

You'll need to think about the times of day you'll be eating and snacking, and when and how you'll provide what you eat. Whether you cook from scratch or get prepackaged items at the store, both calories and portions to be eaten must be considered.

A regular exercise plan or other ways of burning more calories should be implemented. Finding a buddy is also strongly advised. Once you have more experience with the diet and you know what it is you want to accomplish, and how you are getting along, you can set more accurate time lines for what you should be doing when, and when different results should show up.

You will need to find effective ways to shop, prepare snacks, and eat at restaurants and in groups, such as a family gathering. It would also serve you well to learn about how the time of year will effect what you eat, as well as slippery slopes and pitfalls.

All along the way it pays to review your plans and revise them when appropriate. Review your journal and learn from your mistakes as you go along. Don't forget the three-week habit replacement technique! It will serve you well.

Stay aware of your environment, including the other people around you. Find ways to have fun with the diet. One thing vital to making this both a worthwhile and enjoyable trip, is to celebrate your successes. Not merely as they happen, but by reviewing your journal from time to time so that you can remember them, see how far you're getting, and be proud of your progress. And do be proud of yourself! You've earned it and deserve such pride!

Sadly, many people don't succeed on traditional diets, or if they do, they regain their weight once they stop dieting. Some studies suggest that diets don't work, but the people who fail generally blame themselves. This book has listed some common slippery slopes and pitfalls, which have been taken from both diets themselves and problems people encounter as they diet. This list can be an invaluable tool for you in completing your diet if you remember the saying, "Forewarned is forearmed," and review the list often. The value of such reviews is not merely to spot problems that are creeping up as the plan progresses, but to see just how many slippery slopes and pitfalls you have already conquered and make clear how close you are getting to your goals.

If you let it, the RMR diet will change who you are. Who I am now is a person who eats slowly. I am also a person who has a nutritional diet, who eats smaller meals and snacks often, who is happy with what I weigh and how I look, and who is healthier.

Every part of this book has tips and information, and all of them have contributed to bring about yet another landmark for me. That landmark was eventually achieving everything I was hoping for when I first went on the RMR diet. Just as important in this landmark, the devils that used to plague me before I began the RMR diet no longer seem to exist.

Only our memories of yesterday give us the illusion that it still exists. Tomorrow is not here yet. All we have are the slices of now that we call today. Everything you do is done in those slices of now. As each now is conquered, you will move forward and have no need to look back. Now is the time to begin implementing all that you are capable of accomplishing.

About the
Author

Fred Civish is a professional journalist living in Ogden, Utah. He has written more than a thousand articles for dozens of trade journals. He received a bachelor's degree in journalism and later a master's degree in educational psychology, which led to a position as an associate psychologist at the Utah State Training School for the mentally handicapped.

His broad range of hobbies and interests include such diverse things as parachute jumping and diving for abalone in the Pacific.